So you're having

Heart Cath and Angioplasty

Includes peripheral angioplasty

So you're having

Heart Cath

and Angioplasty

MAGNUS OHMAN MD
GAIL COX RN
STEPHEN FORT MD
VICTORIA K. FOULGER RN

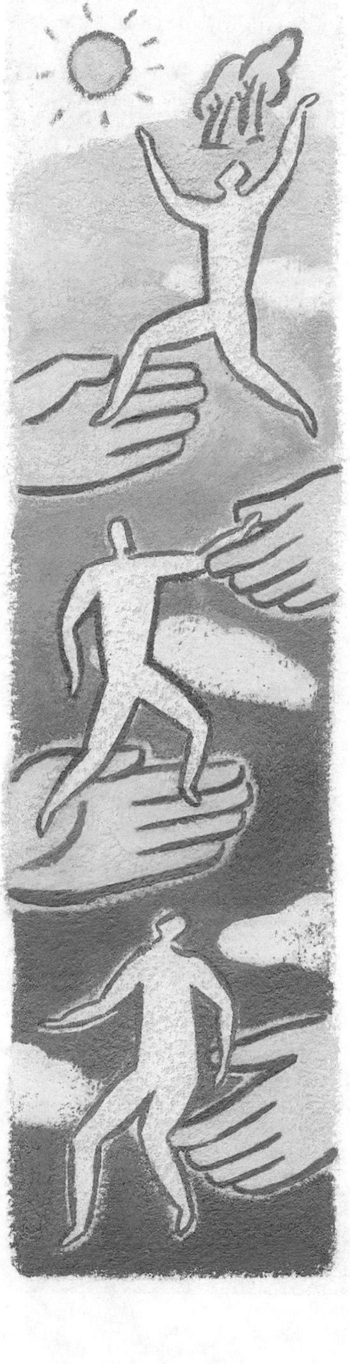

WILEY

BS

Published by John Wiley & Sons, Inc., 111 River Street, Hoboken, NJ 07030

First published in Canada in a somewhat different form by SCRIPT Medical Press, Inc. in 2001

Library of Congress Cataloguing-in-Publication Data
So you're having heart cath and angioplasty / by Stephen Fort ... [et al.].
p. cm.
Based on: So you're having angioplasty / Stephen Fort, Victoria Foulger.
Toronto : SCRIPT Medical Press, 2001.
Includes bibliographical references and index.
ISBN 0-470-83343-2 (pbk.)
1. Coronary heart disease--Popular works. 2. Angioplasty--Popular works. 3. Cardiac catheterization--Popular works. I. Fort, Stephen, 1960- So you're having angioplasty. II. Fort, Stephen, 1960-
RC685.C6S5777 2003
617.4'13--dc21
2003013396

General Editor and Series Creator: Helen Byrt
Editor: Jenny Lass
Copy Editor: Andrea Knight
Book Design and Typesetting: Brian Cartwright, Angela Bobotsis
Cover Illustration: Ross Paul Lindo
Author Photographs: Doug Nicholson, Media Source; University of North Carolina Medical Illustration; Melissa Deschamps
Book Illustrations: Zane Waldman, Bernie Freedman
Publishing Consultant: Malcolm Lester & Associates

Photograph on page 26 courtesy of Media Source; photographs on pages 55, 58 and 133 courtesy of JOMED Canada Inc. (some devices are not approved for use in the U.S.); photographs on page 64 (FLEXI-CUT™) and 67 courtesy of Guidant Corporation; photographs on pages 64 (Rotablator®) and 68 courtesy of Boston Scientific Corporation; photographs on page 65 courtesy of Possis Medical, Inc.; photograph on page 66 courtesy of Cordis Corporation; photograph on page 69 courtesy of Medtronic, Inc.; photograph on page 135 courtesy of CryoVascular Systems. Rotablator® is a registered trademark of Boston Scientific Corporation or its affiliates; CYPHER™ is a registered trademark of Cordis Corporation; Cutting Balloon™ is a trademark of IVT, Inc.; AngioJet® is a registered trademark of Possis Medical, Inc. or its affiliates; PolarCath™ CryoPlasty™ System is a registered trademark of CryoVascular Systems or its affiliates.

The publisher has made every effort to obtain permissions for use of copyrighted material in this book; any errors or omissions will be corrected in the next printing.

Printed and bound in Canada
10 9 8 7 6 5 4 3 2 1

2/11/04

To Alexander Kai, Stephanie, Callan, and our parents.
— S.F. and V.F.

To Elspeth, Edward, Elsa Maria, and Henry,
for their continued support.
—M.O.

To Christian, Michael, Jared, Mom and Dad.
—G.C.

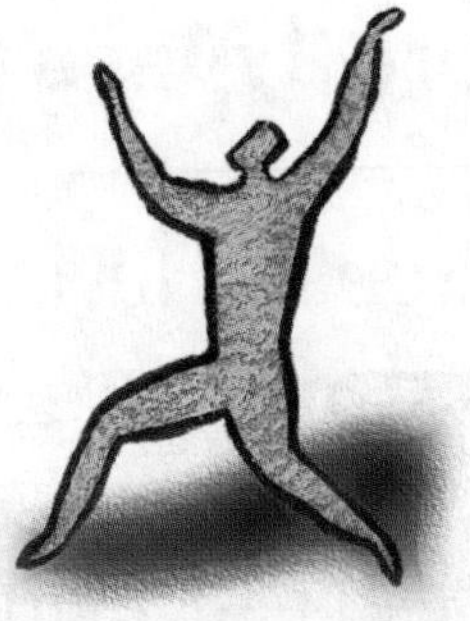

[FORTHCOMING BOOKS *in the* SERIES]

So You're Having
Heart Bypass Surgery

So You're Having
Prostate Surgery

So You're Having A
Hysterectomy

acknowledgments

THIS BOOK WOULD NOT HAVE BEEN POSSIBLE WITHOUT SOME GREAT individuals. First of all, we would like to thank Stephen Fort and Victoria Foulger from Canada who put this idea in motion. We would also like to thank Helen Byrt for her insightful editing of the text. Finally, we would like to thank all of our patients and colleagues—nurses, technicians, and physicians—at Duke University Medical Center and the University of North Carolina (UNC) Heart Center for giving us the insight to provide this text for future patients.

—Magnus Ohman and Gail Cox

THE CREATORS OF HEART CATH AND ANGIOPLASTY ARE unreservedly grateful to many individuals who became caught up in the concept and paid the price with their time and enthusiasm. Early support from Murray Maynard, Joel Rochon, Dana Andrea, and Michelle Lemme made the series possible. Jenny Lass, Malcolm Lester, and Michele George were always there with unwavering optimism. Dr. Stuart McCluskey, Celina Ainsworth, and Kathy Camelon generously shared their hard-won expertise. Thanks are also owed to Andrea Knight, Brian Cartwright, Carol Thomas, Harold Lass, and Angela Bobotsis for creativity and hard work, and Dana Habib, Martha Schutz, Donald Lo, Emma, Annie, Martha, and Milo for reasons they know. Finally we acknowledge with gratitude the patients and families who so willingly shared their road with us: Arni Cohn, the late Robert (Bobby) Frew, Mrs. Joyce Frew, Bill Hogarth, Dr. T. Hofmann, and William Brumitt. Many thanks to you all.

—Helen Byrt

disclaimer

THE INFORMATION PROVIDED IN THIS BOOK MAY NOT apply to all patients, all clinical situations, all hospitals, or all eventualities, and is not intended to be a substitute for the advice of a qualified physician or other medical professional. Always consult a qualified physician about anything that affects your health, especially before starting an exercise program or using a complementary therapy not prescribed by your doctor.

The publisher and the authors make no representations or warranties with respect to the accuracy or completeness of the contents of this work and specifically disclaim all warranties, including without limitation any implied warranties of fitness for a particular purpose. No warranty may be created or extended by any promotional statements. Neither the publisher nor the authors shall be liable for any damages arising herefrom.

contents

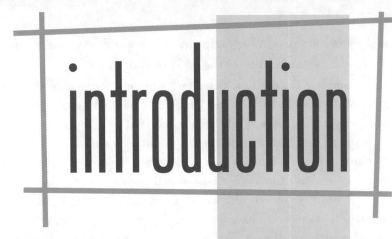

introduction

CARDIAC CATHETERIZATION (HEART CATH) AND ANGIOPLASTY ARE now the most common invasive cardiac procedures that patients undergo in the United States and worldwide. In this book, our aim is to share with you important information about heart cath and angioplasty, including what to expect beforehand and many of the most common questions and answers that we have found, over a decade of practice, to be on most patients' minds. We hope that this book is of great help to you and your loved ones so that you can have a better understanding of the complex nature of percutaneous coronary revascularization—a fancy word for treating your blocked arteries.

Coronary angioplasty, which is also called **percutaneous transluminal coronary angioplasty (PTCA)** or **percutaneous coronary intervention (PCI)**, is an excellent treatment option for most patients with angina and is also becoming increasingly important in the treatment of acute heart attacks. It does not refer to a single operation on your blood vessel, but to many different types of techniques that involve placing a tube (or **catheter**) in your artery to improve the blood flow. Some techniques are more suitable to treat certain blockages than others, and some are more successful than others. In this book you will find several chapters covering all the devices and techniques available to your physician. Our aim is not to make you nervous, but to help you understand why a particular technique is—or is not—being used in your case.

To complete the picture, Chapter 5 will help you decide whether angioplasty is right for you and Chapter 12 will help you to decide whether your angioplasty has been successful.

Just as a combination of factors contributed to your heart disease, a combination of treatments is the most effective way to treat it. As clinicians, we are only too aware that no medical intervention can work by itself. A healthy diet, regular exercise, smoking cessation, and complementary therapies also have a part to play in enabling you to take control of your heart disease. Self-help shouldn't just be an afterthought: it is the core of your treatment, so we have devoted a substantial chapter to strategies that you can use to help yourself (Chapter 11). The most important thing for you to remember is that coronary artery disease is a chronic condition in which you and your significant others must be partners in reducing the risk for further coronary events. Fortunately, combining lifestyle changes with the minimally invasive approach of angioplasty will make your coronary artery disease a condition that can be treated swiftly and efficiently, and allow you to improve your health very quickly.

You are in charge of your health, and never more so than with cardiovascular disease. Your physician can advise and treat you, but the health of your heart is, ultimately, in your hands. Only you can decide which treatment to have, and only you can make the lifestyle changes that will put you on a road to better health. We hope that this book will equip you with the knowledge to make the decisions that are right for you.

Good luck!

Magnus Ohman MD
Gail Cox RN
Stephen Fort MD
Victoria Foulger RN

Chapter 1

coronary artery disease and you

What Happens in this Chapter

- The facts on coronary artery disease
- The likely reasons you have clogged arteries
- The symptoms of angina and a heart attack
- How you can take control of your future

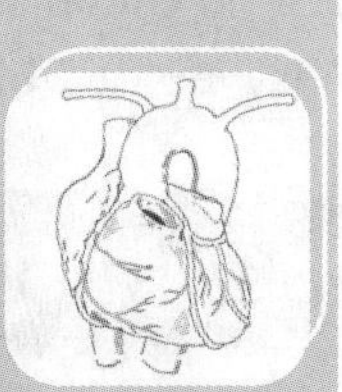

Your heart is a pump the size of your fist. It beats about 60 times a minute to keep blood circulating through your body, carrying nutrients and oxygen to your tissues. It is made of a unique type of muscle called ***myocardium****—the only muscle in the body that keeps contracting without needing a break. The blood supply that allows the myocardium to do this comes from the coronary arteries. When the coronary arteries get blocked by disease, the blood supply to the myocardium is interrupted, resulting in angina or a heart attack. The goal of your heart cath procedure is to find out where the blockages are, so that your physician can decide on the best treatment to restore a normal blood flow to the myocardium.*

How the Heart Works

THE HUMAN HEART IS AN AMAZING PIECE OF ENGINEERING. It is actually two pumps in one: the right half of the heart pumps blood to the lungs to pick up oxygen, while the left half receives the oxygen-rich blood from the lungs and pumps it onward, around the rest of the body. Valves inside the heart keep the blood moving in the right direction and a thin, lubricated membrane outside (called the **pericardium**) ensures that the pumping heart can move easily.

The heart muscle itself (the myocardium) needs a good blood supply to keep contracting, especially during exercise or exertion. The arteries that supply the heart muscle with blood are called the coronary arteries—so-called because from above they look like a crown. The coronary arteries branch off the **aorta** (the main blood vessel in your body) at the point where the oxygen-rich blood leaves the heart, so the heart muscle is the first organ in your body to receive oxygenated blood.

Coronary Artery Disease

Coronary artery disease is a condition in which one or more of the coronary arteries becomes narrowed, so that the heart muscle does not receive enough oxygen. Both angina and heart attacks are usually caused by coronary artery disease, which is the leading cause of death in developed countries.

Coronary artery disease is a form of **atherosclerosis**—a process where the arteries gradually clog up like old water pipes. Over several decades, cholesterol, calcium, and other substances build up under the artery's inner lining, creating a blockage that starts to restrict the flow of blood down the artery (see Figure 1–1). The technical term for this blockage is a **plaque.**

Figure 1–1. How a Plaque Develops

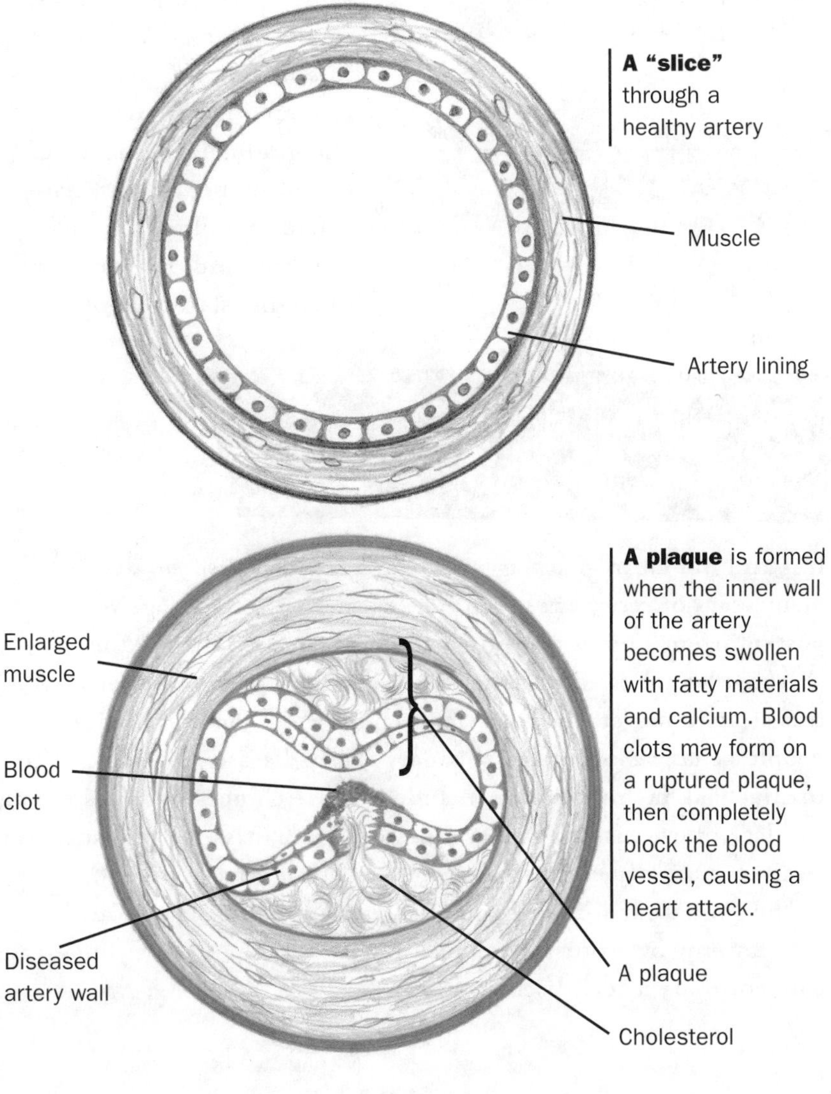
A "slice"
through a
healthy artery
Muscle
Artery lining
Enlarged
muscle
Blood
clot
Diseased
artery wall
A plaque is formed when the inner wall of the artery becomes swollen with fatty materials and calcium. Blood clots may form on a ruptured plaque, then completely block the blood vessel, causing a heart attack.
A plaque
Cholesterol

> "We were staying in a hotel and my husband went to a meeting, so I was alone, and suddenly, as I was walking on the beach, I got very, very bad angina. Somehow I made it back to my chair and waited for my husband. I knew something had happened...I was so weak."
>
> **Mrs. C.V.**

Plaques can become surprisingly large before they start to restrict blood flow because, at first, the artery does its best to compensate for the blockage by stretching and expanding its outer wall. However, this so-called "positive remodeling" has its limits, and gradually the inside of the artery becomes so narrowed that blood flow is reduced, and the symptoms of angina start to appear.

Why Do You Have Coronary Artery Disease?

It is still not clear what triggers coronary artery disease, despite many years of research. It can start as early as the teenage years: post-mortem studies on young soldiers who died during the Vietnam War showed that they had early signs of atherosclerosis. It is clear, however, that there are a number of factors that increase people's chances of getting coronary artery disease—so-called **cardiac risk factors.** These include lifestyle choices such as smoking and lack of exercise, as well as "unmodifiable" risk factors, such as a family history of heart disease (see Key Point box on page 5).

The good news is that if you change the risk factors in your life you can improve your future health considerably, even if you already have coronary artery disease.

[KEY POINT]

Major risk factors for coronary artery disease

Nothing is certain in life, but if you have one or more of these risk factors, then you are more likely to develop coronary artery disease. The more severe the risk factor, the more severe your coronary artery disease is likely to be.

- Family history
- Hyperlipidemia (e.g., high blood cholesterol)
- Smoking
- Diabetes
- High blood pressure
- Obesity
- Sedentary lifestyle

Angina

Usually, the first sign of coronary artery disease is **angina**, a chest pain that starts during exercise and gets better during rest. Most commonly, angina feels like a dull, heavy, constricting sensation that starts in the center of the chest and may spread into the throat or down one arm.

Angina happens when there is an inadequate supply of blood to the myocardium. The heart muscle becomes starved of oxygen and toxins build up, causing cramp-like pain, although there is no permanent damage to the heart muscle. It is also called **myocardial**

ischemia—literally, a reduction of blood to the heart muscle. Angina usually appears first during physical exercise or emotional stress because the heart is beating faster and more strongly, and requires more oxygen.

Figure 1–2. The Heart and Coronary Arteries

These small but crucial arteries supply blood (and oxygen) to the muscle of the heart itself. There are three main arteries—the **right coronary artery** and the two branches of the left coronary artery (the **left anterior descending artery** and the **circumflex artery**).

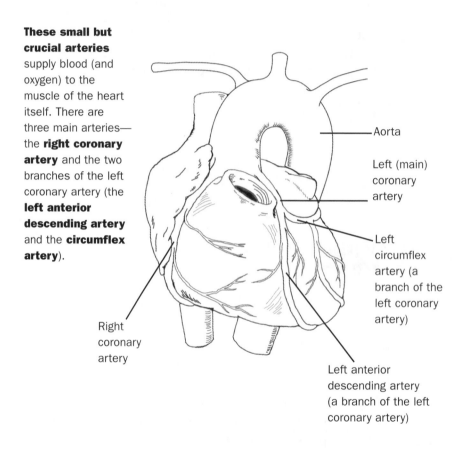

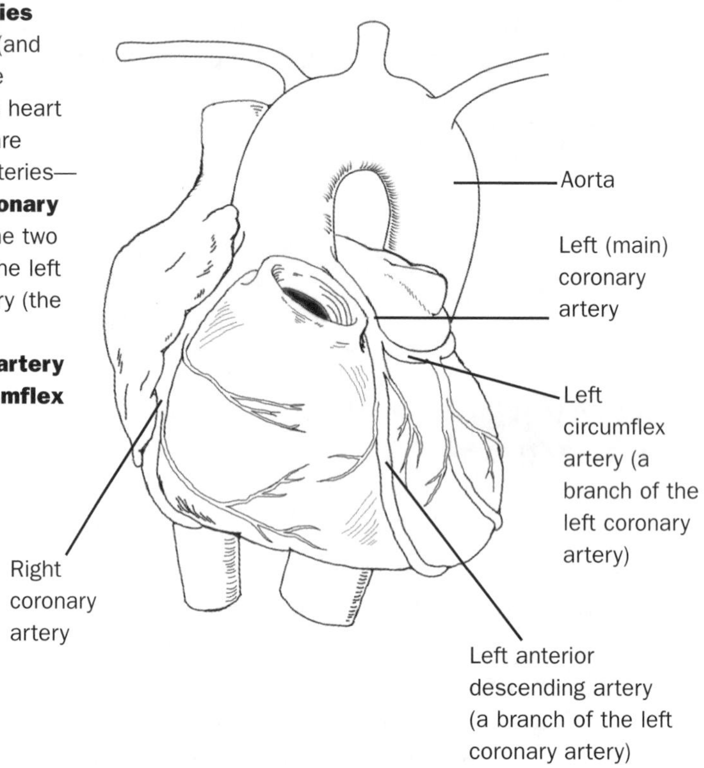

If the blockages in the coronary arteries become severe, angina may be experienced even when resting. This is called **unstable angina**, and is a serious condition: a small number of patients who develop this form of severe angina are likely to have a heart attack within the next few weeks or months.

Not everyone feels pain with angina. "Painless" angina (also known as **silent ischemia**) can show up on an **electrocardiogram,** or **ECG** (see Glossary), although the patient may be unaware of it or experience it as a non-painful symptom such as breathlessness. Silent ischemia is more common than was previously thought, and it may be due to shorter, or less severe, episodes of ischemia than those causing typical angina symptoms. Silent ischemia is treated in the same way as typical angina.

Although angina is most commonly caused by coronary artery disease, it can occasionally result from other heart conditions, for instance a disease of the heart valve called **aortic stenosis** (see Glossary).

A Heart Attack

In angina, blood still flows down the coronary artery and some oxygen reaches the heart muscle. By contrast, in a heart attack (or **myocardial infarction**), the coronary artery is blocked very suddenly and completely, causing a small area of muscle to die and a scar to form. The symptoms of a heart attack are usually different from the symptoms of angina (see Key Point box on page 8).

"Back in 1965 we didn't even know there was such a thing as angina. I think my Mum had it, but they all thought 'pleurisy'—nobody spoke about angina. Father had a coronary thrombosis, too, so it does run in the family."

Robert (Bobby) Frew

"When I had my heart attack it was the first indication of any heart problem. I had some shortness of breath, but never made the connection."

Arni Cohn

Many heart attacks occur in people with no previous warning signs of angina. In addition, up to one-quarter of heart attacks are "silent," without any chest discomfort. The cause of such silent heart attacks is currently unknown. However, since they are more common in people with diabetes—who often have damaged nerves—one theory is that silent heart attacks may result from abnormalities in the nerves that supply the heart, so people simply don't feel the discomfort.

Every chest pain is not angina or a heart attack. There can be many other reasons for chest discomfort, for instance indigestion or pneumonia. Always see your physician if you experience pains in your chest.

[KEY POINT]

If you have the following symptoms you are more likely to be having a heart attack than angina

- Severe, heavy, crushing pain in your chest
- Pain that lasts more than 20 to 30 minutes
- Pain that does not go away when you rest
- No relief from sublingual nitroglycerine
- Breathlessness
- Nausea and, sometimes, vomiting
- Fainting or lightheadedness
- Rapid heartbeat
- Pallor and sweating

If you think you are having a heart attack, dial 911 right away. Do not waste time calling your cardiologist or family doctor.

If you have coronary artery disease, it is likely that you also have atherosclerosis in other arteries of your body. This means that you are at greater risk of having a stroke or poor circulation in other vital organs such as your kidneys. But don't despair. The future is in your hands. Remember, only one cardiac risk factor can't be altered—your family history. Everything else can be changed and it is never too early or too late to start. For advice on what you can do to help yourself, see Chapter 11.

> "Learn as much as you can about what's going on. It helps a lot if you know what they're doing and don't be afraid to ask questions."
>
> **William Brumitt**

What Happens Next?

If your physician thinks you have angina, there are a number of ways to confirm that you have it, find out the reason for it, and decide how serious it is. You may be sent for "non-invasive" tests such as a **treadmill test**, a **nuclear perfusion scan**, or an **echocardiogram** (see Glossary for details of these tests), which will show how well your heart is working. You may then be sent for a **heart cath**, an "invasive" test that involves placing a tube (catheter) into your body to see what state your coronary arteries are in. This procedure is covered in Chapter 4. Your physician may also prescribe lipid-lowering medication at this stage to slow down the progression of atherosclerosis throughout your body, ASA (Aspirin) to reduce the risk of having a heart attack by thinning the blood, and anti-anginal drugs to relieve your angina symptoms.

> "They told me I had 15 percent damage. I found it hard to accept that my heart won't regenerate, grow back like fingernails or skin, but you have to accept it. You have to look at what is behind you, what you want to do in front of you, and plan."
>
> **Arni Cohn**

Chapter 2

getting ready for your heart cath

What Happens in this Chapter

- Tests you'll need before your heart cath
- Consent
- Questions you may want to ask

Preparing for your heart cath not only involves hospital tests and procedures, but also things that you can do for yourself. This is a good time to read up on your procedure so that you can prepare any questions you may wish to ask before you sign the consent form. You can also use the time to make practical arrangements for your hospital visit.

Pre–Heart Cath Tests

A SMALL NUMBER OF BLOOD TESTS AND AN ECG are usually performed before your heart cath. These blood tests include checking to see how your kidneys are working and whether you are anemic. A sample of blood will also be taken and held in reserve in case you need a blood transfusion during or following your heart cath or angioplasty. This blood sample will be used to match donor blood to you, in the unlikely event of an emergency.

> "Before the angioplasty they offered me counseling to help me cope. I refused it—it's normal to be having these problems at age 71."
>
> **Mrs. C.V.**

Pre–Heart Cath Arrangements

The amount of time you will need off work for your heart cath depends partly on how physically demanding your occupation is. If it involves heavy or strenuous exercise, you will need at least 7 days off, particularly if you have your heart cath via your groin. This approach reduces the chance of further bleeding or bruising at the incision site when you do return to work. If your job is fairly sedentary, it may be safe for you to return to work

> [KEY POINT]
>
> **You may not be able to get insurance** to fly until at least 3 months after your procedure if you have an angioplasty. Bear this in mind when booking your heart cath, if you are given a choice of dates.

"I wasn't at all worried because my husband had already had angioplasty twice. I knew about the procedure and I also had 100 percent faith in my doctor."

Mrs. C.V.

as early as the day after you are released from the hospital, if you wish. You can also get back to work faster if you are having your heart cath via your wrist. Bear in mind, too, that you will not be able to drive for a few days after your heart cath, so this may affect how early you can return to work.

If the heart cath findings result in the performance of an angioplasty procedure, your recovery time may be the same. However, your physician will advise you how long you will need off work.

Some patients like to tidy up their paperwork at home before coming into the hospital for their heart cath. Sorting out financial loose ends and updating your will are some suggestions. These kinds of preparations give many people a sense of comfort. While this may or may not be right for you, it is worth considering.

Although this is not specifically related to heart cath, some patients also like to draw up a "living will." A living will clearly informs your family and your physician about exactly what you would like to have happen, and, probably more importantly, would *not* like, in case you fall into a coma. Again, you may not wish to pursue this; it is just something to think about.

Consent

Before you have your heart cath, you will need to give your written consent. This is one of the most important steps of your procedure.

What Exactly Is "Consent"?

You make decisions to take risks every day of your life. Some kind of risk is involved when you cross a road, place a bet on a horse, drive your car, or board an airplane. However, when you go into the hospital to have an operation, the risk you take feels different because you are allowing somebody else, usually a doctor, to make decisions for you. Nonetheless, it is a risk just like every other part of life. Although the physician will be acting in your best interest, it is still important that you understand exactly what you are giving your permission for, or consent to. You are therefore entitled to know what is going to happen to you, why the procedure is needed, and what the risks are. If you agree to have a heart cath, you have given your consent.

You may be asked for your consent for your heart cath on the day of the procedure or in a pre-admission clinic. Either way, it is an important part of your heart cath experience that can sometimes cause further anxiety and lead to misunderstanding. It is important that you read the consent form carefully and understand what it is you are signing. Do not feel pressured to sign the consent form immediately. If there is enough time you can always take the form

> "The night before they give you something to help you sleep a bit, but I wasn't overly concerned or nervous. They showed me a diagram and there were videos about what they were going to do."
>
> **Bill Hogarth**

[KEY POINT]

Take your time before you sign your consent form.

home and bring it back on the day of your procedure. Most consent forms will have paragraphs in them saying that the physician may carry out additional procedures should the need arise (for example, in an emergency situation).

Ask your physician or the nurse, if you can, what additional procedures may be carried out and what the possible outcomes of these procedures might be. If you are worried about any part of the procedure, or you feel you have not received a clear answer on anything, now is the time to say so. Once you have signed the consent form, it will be assumed that you understand and accept the risks involved.

Risks of a Heart Cath

Because a heart cath involves placing catheters and infusing "dye" into an organ as complex as your heart, there are a number of potential complications—unwanted medical events—that may occur during or after the procedure (see More Detail box on page 16).

Bear in mind that risks are only estimates, and you are unlikely to have any of these complications. Your physician will certainly be doing his or her best to prevent them. The risks associated with your heart cath are affected by the type of blockage you have, the strength (or weakness) of your heart's muscle, and any other medical conditions (for example, asthma or diabetes) that you may have.

Asking Questions

Feel free to ask any questions you like before signing your consent form. Reading up on the procedure beforehand is helpful because you will understand more of what you are being told and be able to come up with questions more easily (see Self Help box on page 15).

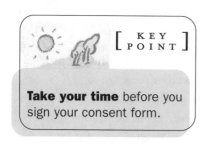

Questions You Might Like to Ask Before Your Heart Cath

- Why do I need a heart cath?
- What will happen if blockages are found in my arteries?
- If I need an angioplasty, will you do it right away or will I need to come back?
- What are the risks?
- How long will it take?
- Will I be awake?
- How long will I stay in the hospital?
- When can I return to work?

The Patient Diary at the back of the book also has space for your questions.

What Happens Next?

Once you have signed the consent form the next step is the heart cath procedure itself.

The Possible Complications of a Heart Cath

[MORE DETAIL]

The main benefit of a heart cath is that it gives a clear picture of your heart disease so that your physician can recommend treatment that is right for you. However, as with all medical procedures, there are risks and you should be aware of these before giving your consent for the procedure (for more on patient consent, see pages 12–14). These rates are estimates and individual situations may vary.

- Severe bleeding or bruising happens in about 1 in 100 people.
- The radio-opaque dye can occasionally lead to allergic reactions (about 4 per 1,000 people) or deterioration in the function of your kidneys (especially in people with pre-existing kidney disease).
- It is not common, but there may be infection, pain, or blockage of the blood vessel at the site of the puncture.
- Very occasionally the catheters can damage one of the heart's blood vessels, or, in about 4 per 1,000 people, cause a stroke. There is a risk of a stroke or mini-stroke in about 7 per 10,000 people.
- Angina can occur during the procedure. If it does, inform the nurse and cardiologist immediately.
- One in 100 people suffer abnormal heartbeats during the procedure.
- As with all X-rays, there is exposure to radiation. One coronary angiogram is equivalent to approximately fifteen trans-Atlantic flights.
- Rarely, some people suffer a heart attack or die during or after the procedure. However, this occurs in fewer than 1 in 1,000 people.

The risks described above are based on information published in the ACC/AHA guidelines for coronary angiography in May 1999.

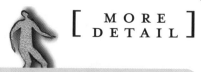

Chapter 3

the day of your heart cath

What Happens in this Chapter

- Making a hospital checklist
- Arrival at the hospital
- Tips for friends and family
- Transfer to the cath lab

Finally, the day arrives when you will have the procedure. It is normal for you to feel anxious but good preparation helps. When you get to the hospital you will be assigned a bed and a nurse to look after you. There will be some routine tests and you may be given a mild sedative. You will then be taken to the ***cardiac catheterization laboratory (cath lab)*** *where your heart cath will be carried out.*

Planning Your Day

You will probably be one of a number of patients undergoing the same procedure that day. Although the heart cath procedure takes less than 1 hour, you will probably be in the hospital for 6 to 8 hours in total. However, you will be discharged the same day you have the procedure. If you receive angioplasty, this additional procedure will take 30 minutes to 4 hours and you will stay in the hospital overnight. Be sure to pack everything you need to stay in the hospital overnight in case you have an angioplasty, including all of your medications. Remember to make

[SELF-HELP]

Hospital Checklist

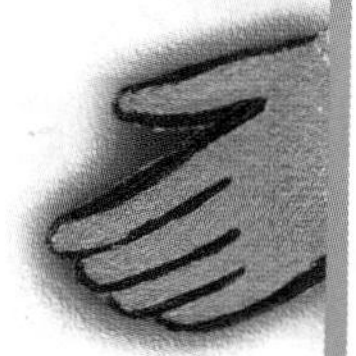

This checklist may be useful before you leave for the hospital:

- Do not eat or drink anything for 6 hours prior to arriving at the hospital except your medications. ○
- Take ALL your medications with a sip of water. ○
- Blood-thinning medication such as Coumadin should have been stopped 3 to 5 days before your procedure, unless you were specifically told to continue by your physician. ○
- Bring in your daily medications (in their bottles). ○
- Pack an overnight bag that includes pajamas, slippers, and toiletries. ○
- Bring some reading material with you, but forget about work or business material. Sedative medication during your procedure will make you drowsy afterward and unable to concentrate on work. ○

arrangements to be taken home from the hospital because you will be advised not to drive home yourself.

While the exact arrangements vary from hospital to hospital, you are likely to be asked to follow these instructions prior to your heart cath:

> "Make sure what pain medications they're going to use and whether or not you're allergic to them in any way."
>
> **William Brumitt**

- Don't eat or drink anything for 6 hours before arriving at the hospital.
- Inform the person scheduling your heart cath if you are allergic to contrast dye or shellfish.
- Arrive at the hospital and report to the cath lab or an area otherwise specified by your physician.
- Bring your regular medications in their bottles with you.
- You will be given special instructions if you are taking medication for diabetes, or if you are taking blood thinners such as Coumadin.

Arrival in the Hospital

When you arrive at the hospital, you will register at the cath lab and be brought back to a holding area. After you have changed into a hospital gown, a nurse will weigh you, check your vital signs, and insert an intravenous line into one of your arms. This will be used to give you fluids and to administer drugs during and after your procedure. You will then be examined by a physician and your consent for the operation

> "I was transferred from one hospital to another and it was the next day that they did the heart cath."
>
> **William Brumitt**

will be obtained (see pages 12–14). Your groin will be shaved, and routine blood tests will be performed to check that your kidneys are working properly and that you are not anemic. An ECG will also be performed. You may have already gone through some of these steps on previous hospital visits.

While you are waiting for your heart cath, there will be a nurse assigned to look after you (and a number of other patients). Now is the time to tell the nurse about any anxieties or unanswered questions you have.

[KEY POINT]

If you are on oral anticoagulants, e.g., warfarin (Coumadin), or diabetes medication, e.g., metformin (Glucophage), you must tell your physician or clinic before you go for your heart cath. Warfarin is normally discontinued for 3 to 5 days before a heart cath to reduce the risk of heavy bleeding from the wound site. Metformin is discontinued before a heart cath because it may cause a build-up of lactic acid in the blood, which is a serious condition that can be fatal.

[SELF-HELP]

Back problems

Backache is a particularly common complaint from many patients after a heart cath and can make the recovery period even more uncomfortable. If you have back problems, tell your physician BEFORE you go into the cath lab.

Transfer to the Cardiac Catheterization Laboratory (Cath Lab)

Unless you are the first case of the day, the exact time of your procedure can only be estimated; there is no guarantee when it will start or finish. While your nursing staff and doctors will do their best to give you some idea of when your procedure will take place, this will be affected by how long other patients' heart caths take (which can be difficult to estimate) and whether there are any unexpected emergencies.

For more about arrival at the cath lab, and getting comfortable, see Chapter 4.

"They explained pretty thoroughly what they were going to do. They said they may find the need to put in a stent, depending upon what they found when they went in."

William Brumitt

Friends and Family

Depending on individual hospital policy, your friends and family members may be allowed to stay with you before your heart cath. This often helps to calm anxiety and will give you support when you're asking questions during the process of giving your consent.

Family and friends will not be allowed to stay with you after your transfer to the cath lab. During your heart cath, there is often a special waiting area for friends and family. If they do not want to remain in the waiting area, suggest to them that they leave details of how they can be contacted with the nursing staff, in the event that a member of your medical team wishes to speak with them. Because you may also have an angioplasty, and the time required for this procedure can vary greatly—from 30 minutes to 4 hours—no guarantee can be given about when you will be transferred back to the ward.

What Happens Next?

Once you are in the cath lab, your heart cath can begin.

Chapter 4

the heart cath procedure

What Happens in this Chapter

- Why a heart cath is needed
- What is a heart cath?
- Step-by-step guide to heart cath
- The risks
- Decoding your X-ray pictures — and your diagnosis

A heart cath can help you and your medical team get the inside story on your heart. By injecting a special dye into the arteries of your heart and looking at the X-ray pictures of your blood vessels on a TV screen in real time, your cardiologist can see which arteries are blocked, where, and how badly. This will help him or her to decide whether you need angioplasty, bypass surgery, or just more drug therapy.

Why a Heart Cath is Needed

IN ORDER FOR YOUR PHYSICIAN TO HAVE A CLEAR understanding of your heart condition, he or she needs to access the most likely cause of the problem—your coronary arteries. A technique called **cardiac catheterization**, or a heart cath, lets your cardiologist get as close as possible to your heart without having to open up your chest.

What is a Heart Cath?

During a heart cath, tubes called catheters are inserted into the arteries of your heart through the groin or arm so that your physician can perform valuable tests and procedures (see Figure 4–1, page 24). One of these tests involves taking X-ray pictures of your coronary arteries. Doctors call this X-ray test **coronary angiography**. It is the most useful information that you and your medical team could have.

Blood vessels don't normally show up on X-rays, so the pictures are created by injecting a dye that is visible to X-rays (radio-opaque) into the blood vessels of the heart. The physician then uses the X-ray machine to guide him or her through the procedure and record the pictures. There are three main coronary arteries that supply blood to the heart muscle (see Figure 1–2, page 6). During the heart cath, your cardiologist will look at all three of these arteries to check for disease.

After your X-ray pictures are taken, your physician will know the condition of your coronary arteries and can make recommendations on how best to treat you. If your arteries are blocked, you may be offered coronary angioplasty (see Chapter 5). Most likely, your physician will want to go ahead with your angioplasty right away, while your catheter is still in place. For the angioplasty, new tools will be inserted through the catheter, which will be used to widen your blocked arteries.

Figure 4–1. Cardiac Catheterization (A Heart Cath)

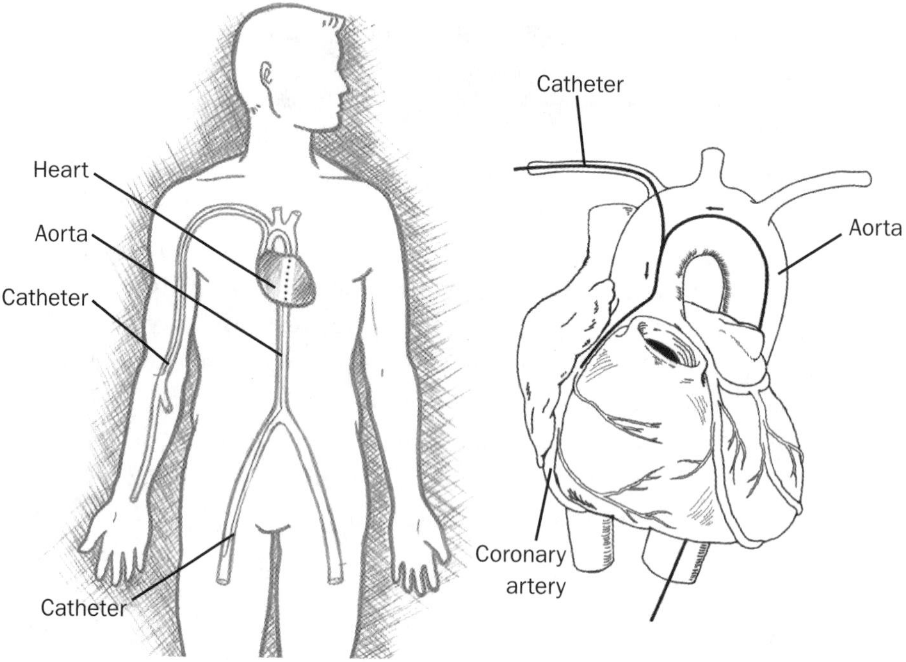

A. **B.**

During a heart cath a tube called a catheter is inserted into the heart's blood vessels via an artery in the arm or the groin (A). The catheter is then used to inject radio-opaque dye and insert angioplasty equipment into the coronary arteries (B).

Your Heart Cath and Angioplasty Procedure

[MORE DETAIL]

The following are the basic steps of your heart cath.

1. You are given a local anesthetic injection into the skin above a blood vessel in your groin or arm.
2. A small incision is made through the skin and a needle is inserted into the blood vessel.
3. A **sheath** (short plastic tube) is placed into the blood vessel and a catheter (long thin tube) is inserted into it.
4. The catheter is passed all the way to your coronary arteries.
5. Radio-opaque dye is injected into the coronary arteries.
6. X-ray pictures of your arteries are taken.

This is what will happen if you go on to have an angioplasty:

1. You are given blood-thinning medication.
2. A **guide wire** is passed through the catheter and into the narrowed region of your coronary artery ("wiring the vessel").
3. The angioplasty balloon travels along the wire into the narrowed blood vessel.
4. The balloon is inflated and deflated to widen the artery.
5. A **stent** (small supporting tube) is placed in the artery, if required.
6. Other procedures are performed, if required.
7. The incision is closed.

The Cath Lab

When you reach the cardiac catheterization laboratory (or cath lab) you will be introduced to all the staff. In addition to your physician, there will be nurses and technicians, and, possibly, a junior physician. The staffing arrangements will vary from hospital to hospital. One of the first things you may notice is the temperature. The temperature inside modern cath labs is deliberately kept low to ensure reliable running of the X-ray and recording equipment. Since you will be wearing a thin gown, you may feel a little uncomfortable until you are settled on the X-ray table and covered in sterile drapes.

The table is narrow and not designed with comfort in mind, but try to make yourself as comfortable as possible. If you need another pillow, ask for one. Although a heart cath is a relatively short procedure (under an hour, compared to an angioplasty that can sometimes take many hours), your comfort is important. Apart from the fact that cath lab staff want you to be happy, there is also a practical reason for making you comfortable: if you move around a lot it will be harder for the cardiologist to get good pictures.

Figure 4–2. The Cath Lab

The cardiac catheterization laboratory is where you will have your heart cath and, if needed, your angioplasty.

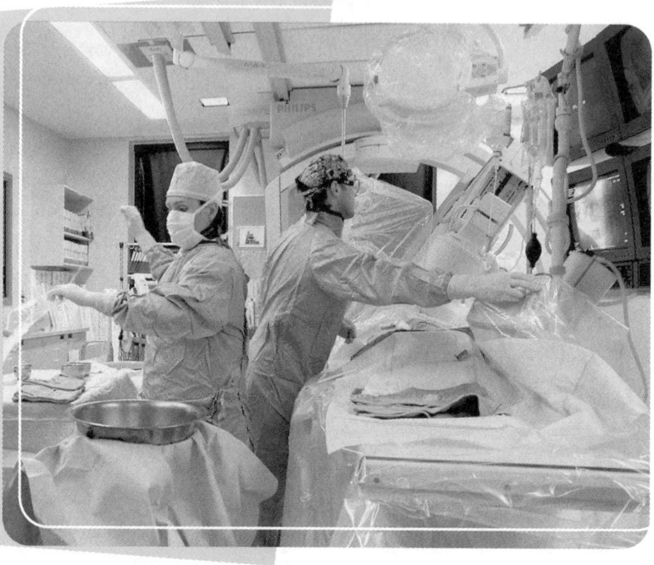

Help Yourself to Better Pictures

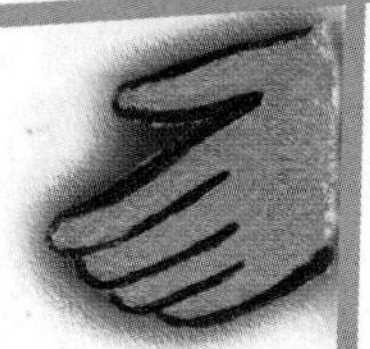

- It is normal to feel anxious, particularly if you are having a heart cath for the first time. It may help to talk to someone else who has had the procedure. Your physician or nurse may be able to put you in touch with someone.
- Make a list of questions that you want to ask your doctor or nurse and take the list with you on the day of your procedure. If you do not understand something you have been told, ask for an explanation. Having a friend or family member with you can help. Do not sign the consent form if you are unhappy about anything.
- Try to ask everything you want to know before you go into the catheterization laboratory because, once the procedure is underway, your medical team will be concentrating on the task at hand.
- Try not to move around to get a better view of the X-ray monitors because your heart will move, spoiling the pictures. The camera will be placed in the best possible position for quick and easy recording. If you can't see properly, ask your physician to show you the pictures at the end.
- If you feel any pain during the procedure, or experience any problems in your arm, leg, or chest afterward, tell the medical team immediately.

Sedatives

Most patients feel a little anxious before their heart cath—this is normal. If you become very anxious, you can ask for a mild sedative. However, your physician may need you to make a decision about your treatment while you are in the cath lab, so the sedative you are given cannot be too strong. Your sedative medication will make you drowsy, but you will still be conscious. The type and dose of sedative medication will vary from hospital to hospital.

Preparing for the Heart Cath

Once you are lying on the X-ray table, the lab staff will attach leads to your chest and legs, just like when you had an electrocardiogram (ECG or EKG). These will allow your heart rate and rhythm to be monitored during the procedure.

The place on your skin where the tubes (or catheters) will be inserted will now be washed with a sterilizing solution to prevent infection. Since most sterilizing solutions contain alcohol, expect the fluid to feel cold. Most cardiologists use the groin to insert the catheters, although your physician may choose to use your arm.

Heart caths using the arm can be done via the wrist (see More Detail box on page 29) or via the inside of the elbow (**brachial**). The brachial technique is quite rare and usually reserved for people with circulation problems in the legs and when the wrist cannot be used for some reason.

You will notice TV screens (monitors) on one side of you. This is where your X-ray pictures will be displayed during your procedure. You will be able to see some, but not all, of the pictures. The X-ray camera in front of your chest will sometimes block your view. Inform your cardiologist if at any stage the X-ray camera comes too close for comfort.

Heart Cath Via Your Wrist [MORE DETAIL]

The technique of carrying out heart caths via the wrist instead of the groin is growing in popularity, although it is still not used by all physicians and is not an option for some patients. Many physicians are not trained for the technique, and it is technically more difficult because the artery used (the radial artery) is much smaller than the one in the groin. With practice, physicians can perform most heart caths equally well via the groin or the wrist.

To see whether you are able to have your heart cath performed this way, the hospital will need to do a simple circulation test called the **Allen's test** (see Glossary). This reveals whether you have one or two open blood vessels in your wrist. You will need two open blood vessels for a wrist heart cath.

The major advantage of a wrist heart cath for the patient is that he or she can sit up immediately after the procedure and will avoid a long period of bed rest—the most uncomfortable feature of heart cath of the groin. The downside for the patient is that the insertion of the sheath can be painful due to the small size of the arteries.

Heart Cath Procedure

The first step of your heart cath is making the incision so that the catheters can enter an artery in your groin or arm. To make the incision more comfortable for you, the cath lab team will "freeze" your skin with an injection of local anesthetic. A small incision is then made into the skin by a scalpel, then a needle and a short tube called a sheath are inserted into your blood vessel. Even after the anesthetic, you may still feel some pulling and pushing in your arm or groin, but it should not be painful.

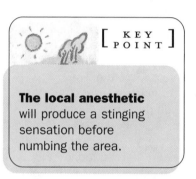

Once the sheath is safely in place, your cardiologist will insert the long catheters all the way to your heart. He or she will place the tips of the catheters in each of your three coronary arteries under X-ray guidance. Radio-opaque dye is then injected into your blood vessels.

When the dye is injected, you may feel a peculiar warm sensation spreading around your body as the dye travels through your blood vessels. Another odd side effect is the feeling that you have passed urine. Do not worry, this is just an illusion and is entirely harmless.

[KEY POINT]

The local anesthetic will produce a stinging sensation before numbing the area.

Any narrowings in the blood vessels will be displayed on the TV monitors, so the cath lab team can record the position and severity of the diseased areas. You have the option of watching the TV monitoring screen to view the procedure or you may choose not to—the choice is yours! Because disease in blood vessels can sometimes affect just one part of the vessel wall without affecting the rest, your physician will need to see different views of your blood vessels. He or she will move the X-ray camera around and take pictures on both sides of your chest.

Because your heart moves with every breath you take, you will be asked to either hold your breath, or take a deep breath, while the pictures are being taken.

The whole procedure takes less than 1 hour and most patients find it relatively easy to tolerate.

[KEY POINT]

The more disease in your blood vessels and the more blood vessels that are affected, the more likely you are to be recommended bypass surgery.

Left Ventricular Angiography

At the beginning or end of your heart cath procedure, another type of catheter, called a **pig-tail catheter**, is often used to look at the muscular pumping action of the heart and the health of the heart valves. This is called a **left ventricular** (or **LV**) **angiogram.**

Right Heart Catheterization

A "regular" heart cath usually enters the left side of the heart. By contrast, **right heart catheterization**, or **Swan-Gantz catheterization**, is used in patients with heart failure (weakened heart) or unexplained shortness of breath. It is used to check the chambers and valves in the right side of the heart, the part of the heart that

"The main discomfort is that you can't move, especially afterward, when, of course, you have to be immobile and your bladder is irritated from the dye. I didn't realize that I should have asked for a bedpan before the nurse put the press on me. I know it's a small thing, but at the time it was very uncomfortable."

Mrs. C.V.

Figure 4–3. X-ray Pictures (Angiograms) of the Coronary Arteries

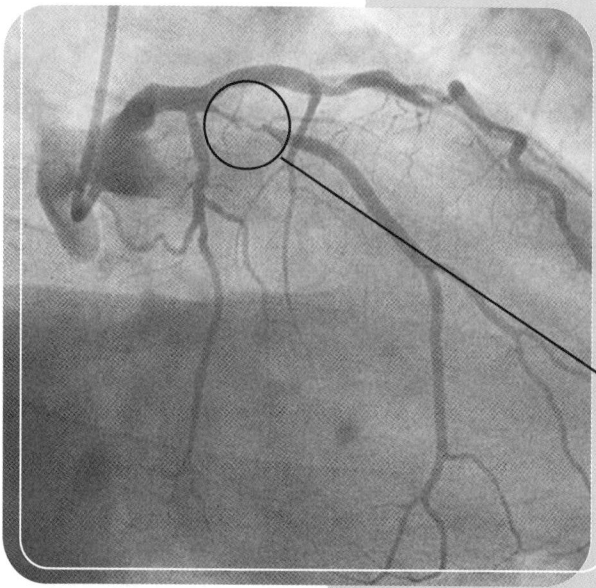

A narrowed artery before angioplasty.

Narrowed artery

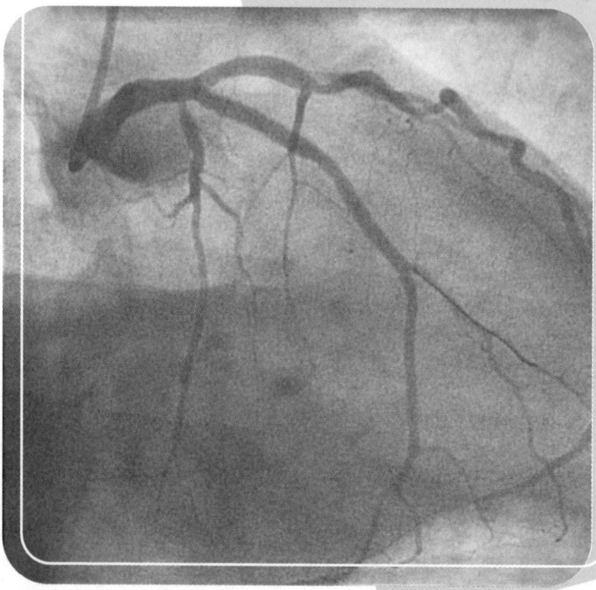

The same artery after a successful angioplasty and stent insertion.

pumps blood to the lungs. It helps the cardiologist better understand the heart function, and provides information to the heart surgeon on any leaky or blocked heart valves.

This procedure usually prolongs the heart cath by 10 to 20 minutes or so. The cardiologist will insert the catheter through a vein instead of an artery—usually the **femoral vein** (in the arm) or, less often, the **jugular vein** (in the neck). It is not usually painful, and although it can result in bleeding problems, the bleeding is generally easy to stop because the blood pressure in the veins is much lower than in arteries.

> "After my angiogram they told me I had a 90 percent blockage in the circumflex artery."
>
> **Mrs. C.V**

Peripheral Angioplasty

At the end of your heart cath, your physician may take the opportunity to check out and treat other arteries he or she suspects are narrowed, such as the arteries in your legs or kidneys. This is called **peripheral angioplasty**. For more detail on this procedure, see Chapter 8.

What Does Your Heart Cath Mean?

Once your heart cath is finished, you will probably be quite anxious to know the results. Your cardiologist will tell you what he or she has seen while you are still in the cath lab (see "Decoding your Diagnosis," page 34).

Decoding your Diagnosis

[MORE DETAIL]

Single-, double-, or triple-vessel disease — Disease in one, two, or three of the coronary arteries (for more on coronary arteries, see Figure 1–2, page 6).

A plaque — The technical term for the blockage in your coronary artery. Plaques are made of cholesterol, scar tissue, and, sometimes, calcium.

Stenosis — A narrowing in a coronary artery, caused by a plaque; classified as mild, moderate, or severe, or expressed as a percentage. An artery can become 70 percent narrowed before symptoms of angina appear. Narrowings of 20 to 50 percent are a sign of early disease, do not necessarily result in angina, and are usually treated with medication and diet.

Left main disease — Disease in the left (main) coronary artery, the most important blood vessel of the heart. If this vessel is severely diseased, bypass surgery is usually recommended, although angioplasty may be possible.

Occlusion — A blockage of the vessel, usually expressed as a percentage (e.g., 50 percent). Chronic occlusions (a blockage over 6 months old) can be very difficult to unblock by angioplasty. Even if successful, the re-narrowing rate after angioplasty is higher. Bypass surgery is often preferred in this situation.

Impaired left ventricular function — The pumping action of the main chamber of the heart (the left ventricle). This is often impaired after a heart attack and can strongly influence whether you undergo angioplasty or bypass surgery.

In general, mild heart disease (less than 50 percent narrowing) of one, two, or three of your blood vessels is usually treated with medication and diet. In moderate disease, where 50 to 70 percent of the artery is blocked, treatment depends on how bad your symptoms are and the results of other cardiac tests. Severe "single-vessel" disease (more than 70 percent narrowing of one blood vessel) is usually treated with angioplasty. Severe "three-vessel" disease is more likely to be treated with bypass surgery.

What Happens Next?

If your doctor discovers that one or more of your arteries are blocked, he or she will recommend whether angioplasty, heart bypass surgery, or medication alone is the best treatment for you while you are still in the cath lab. However, the choice is yours. Even if your physician feels that angioplasty is your best option, you can ask to think about your decision and end the procedure at this point, unless it is an emergency, in which case the physician will probably advise you to go ahead and have the procedure done right there on the spot. If, after you have recovered from your heart cath, you decide that you would like angioplasty after all, you can always ask your doctor to refer you for an angioplasty at a later date. If your physician feels strongly that you need heart bypass surgery, you will be referred to a specialist called a **cardiothoracic surgeon**. For more information on bypass surgery, see the book *So You're Having Heart Bypass Surgery* (details on page 149).

If you agree to have an angioplasty immediately following your heart cath, there will be no break between the heart cath and angioplasty procedures. Because angioplasty is performed through the same incision as your heart cath, you will remain on the X-ray table with the sheath inserted in your arm or groin. Chapter 6 tells you what will happen during your angioplasty.

Chapter 5

is angioplasty right for you?

What Happens in this Chapter

- All about angioplasty and heart bypass surgery
- The risks and benefits of these procedures

Your X-ray pictures will tell your physician whether your coronary arteries are narrowed, and how badly. If your arteries are narrowed, your physician will recommend one of three possible treatments: more medication, angioplasty, or bypass surgery. Knowing the risks and benefits of these options will help you to understand the recommendations that your physician makes and decide which route to recovery is best for you.

The Treatment Decision

Once your Heart Cath and other tests have confirmed that you have narrowed coronary arteries and angina, you and your physician will need to agree on the best treatment. Angina can be treated with either drug therapy, angioplasty, or coronary artery bypass surgery. Your physician will make a recommendation based on his or her past experience with patients whose medical situation is similar to yours, the number of factors in your life that may affect the health of your heart (for example, obesity), whether or not you have any other serious medical or surgical conditions, and his or her knowledge of the most recent scientific studies.

Your state of health may mean that the choice is obvious. For instance, you may have had a heart attack due to a blockage that can easily be cleared with angioplasty, or emergency bypass surgery may be needed. Sometimes the decision is less clear-cut and you will be able to go with your own preference. If there is no particular medical reason to choose one treatment over another, the decision may depend on practical considerations, such as locally available hospital resources and how quickly you need to return to work.

This chapter summarizes the advantages and disadvantages of drug therapy, bypass surgery, and angioplasty, based on the most recently available scientific information. Our intention is to give you enough information to be able to make an informed decision about your treatment. If you prefer to leave the decision-making to your physician, that's fine, too.

"I saw others walking around after their angioplasty and thought, 'It can't be too bad if they're all OK.' Other patients in hospital said it wasn't too bad and it was helpful having someone to talk to. You realize it's a common procedure and lots of other people have it."

Bill Hogarth

How to Decide?

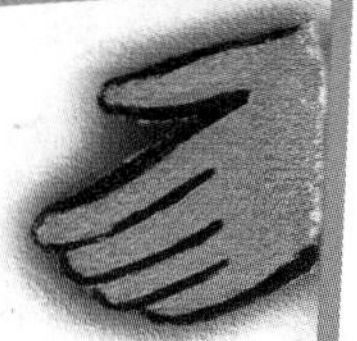

- It is likely that you will be able to have a say in your treatment. However, in an emergency situation, the cardiologist will proceed with the treatment that will best help you.
- Although your health may dictate which treatments are most appropriate for you, it is still worth knowing the pros and cons of your treatment so that you can give fully informed consent.
- Towards the end of your heart cath, it is common for your cardiologist to make treatment recommendations while you are still in the cath lab. If he or she feels that angioplasty is your best option, you can give your consent to having angioplasty done immediately after your heart cath.
- If you wish to think about your treatment options, or angioplasty is not an option that your cardiologist recommends, you can make your decision after you have recovered from your heart cath.
- If you wish, you may get a second opinion from another physician, especially if you have many treatments to choose from.
- Once you have decided on a treatment, you are allowed to change your mind.
- For information on bypass surgery, see the book *So You're Having Heart Bypass Surgery* (details on page 149).

Drug Treatment

All patients with angina are treated with medication, whether they choose to have angioplasty or not. You may be on many drugs, some to relieve your angina, others to reduce the risks of a heart attack, and still others aimed at slowing the progression of your heart disease, including drugs to lower your cholesterol and blood pressure (for a detailed discussion of medications, see Chapter 13).

With the large number of potent and effective anti-angina drugs currently available, many patients with mild or moderate angina can be successfully treated by drug therapy alone. You may choose to simply manage your angina by continuing with, or adding to, your existing medication.

Obviously, the main advantage of treating your angina with medication alone is that you don't have to undergo the pain or inconvenience of a hospital procedure.

The main disadvantage of dealing with your angina by drug treatment alone is the sheer number of medications you may have to take. By contrast, after a successful angioplasty or bypass surgery you *may* be able to cut down on the number of drugs you take because you should no longer need to take medication for your angina symptoms.

The greater the number of drugs you take and the higher their doses, the more likely you are to suffer drug side effects. A list of the common side effects associated with heart medications is given in Chapter 13. It is impossible for your physician to predict whether you will suffer any side effects. Bear in mind, too, that it is impossible for him or her to give any guarantees about how well your angina will respond to medication, or which drug will be most effective. A period of trial and error is often needed before your physician can find the right combination of drugs—and doses—to suit you.

Despite these limitations, drug therapy alone may be the right long-term option for you if you are unhappy about the risks of a hospital procedure and if your angina is well controlled—that is, if your angina attacks are infrequent and you can lead a normal or near-normal life with few or no restrictions.

Remember, if your angina gets worse in the future, you can always change your mind and ask your physician to refer you for angioplasty or bypass surgery.

What is Angioplasty?

[KEY POINT]

If your angina is NOT well controlled by your medication, for example, if you experience angina when doing nothing to provoke an attack, or you suffer recurrent or prolonged episodes of angina, you should tell your doctor.

Angioplasty involves unblocking your narrowed coronary arteries by inserting a small balloon into each artery and inflating the balloon at the site of the blockage. This presses the blockage to the sides of the artery and stretches (dilates) the artery slightly, allowing blood to flow freely once more. It involves making a small incision (cut) in either the arm or the groin to insert the balloon equipment all the way up to the heart. (For more on the angioplasty procedure, see Chapter 6.)

What is Bypass Surgery?

Coronary artery bypass surgery was first reported in 1967 and has since undergone many improvements. A heart surgeon creates a "bypass" around the blocked coronary artery by using a length of blood vessel taken from either the leg or chest. The resulting bypass is called a **coronary artery bypass graft** or **CABG** (pronounced "cabbage"). Thus, bypass surgery does not attempt to unblock the coronary arteries—it simply creates another route for the blood to reach the heart muscle. For more on bypass surgery, see the book, *So You're Having Heart Bypass Surgery*.

"I managed for years on just medication until my bypass, although I was never free from my angina."

Robert (Bobby) Frew

The Advantages of Angioplasty

Simpler Procedure

The main advantage of angioplasty over bypass surgery is that it is quicker and less traumatic. An angioplasty procedure takes on average 1 to 2 hours to perform, depending on the number of blockages and how complicated they are—sometimes even less. You are awake the whole time, and only a small incision in either your groin or arm is involved. This means that you recover fairly quickly. Bypass operations can take 3 to 4 hours to perform, involve opening up your chest, and you may take weeks or months to recover. Not surprisingly, angioplasty is often the choice of people who have major responsibilities at home or work.

No General Anesthetic

Bypass surgery requires a general anesthetic. Angioplasty uses only a local anesthetic injection and a mild sedative injected through the intravenous line in your arm. This means that you avoid the risks of a general anesthetic and your recovery period is much shorter.

No Grafts

Bypass surgery involves grafting a vein or artery from elsewhere in the body onto the heart to bypass the blocked artery. The pieces of vein or artery used for the bypass are called **conduits**. These are usually taken from leg veins or from arteries behind the breastbone. By contrast, angioplasty does not need conduits, so there is less pain and discomfort, and, again, the whole procedure is much simpler. In addition, it is sometimes hard to find suitable conduits in people with medical conditions such as varicose veins or lung disease. Angioplasty does not have these limitations.

Less Chance of a Blood Transfusion

A blood transfusion is rarely needed for coronary angioplasty, but is more common if you undergo bypass surgery. Only in the unlikely situation that you have severe and life-threatening bleeding during angioplasty—for instance, as a result of all the blood-thinning medication you receive—will a blood transfusion be needed.

Shorter Hospital Stay

After routine bypass surgery, patients generally stay in the hospital about 5 days. If all goes well, with an angioplasty, you will be out of the hospital the next day.

Less Risk (for some patients)

Up to 1 in 50 people having bypass surgery suffer a mild stroke. For angioplasty, the risk is about 1 in 200 (for more on risks, see pages 44–47).

Quicker Recovery

Angioplasty is less traumatic than a bypass operation, so the total recovery time (both in the hospital and at home) is shorter. Immediately after bypass surgery you will be transferred, still unconscious, to the intensive care unit. By contrast, after angioplasty, you will be fully conscious and returned to your room or the intensive care unit where you will spend just a few hours in a special recovery area, then go home the next day.

Once home, the site of the incision will take a few days to fully heal, but you should return to normal very quickly. You may take weeks or months to return to normal following bypass surgery.

Angioplasty ***may*** *be a better option for you than bypass surgery if you have*

[MORE DETAIL]

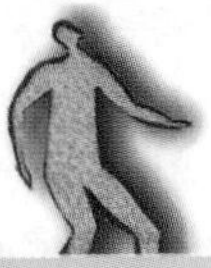

- had a very recent heart attack
- varicose veins
- lung disease (e.g., asthma or bronchitis)
- any medical condition that means you shouldn't have a general anesthetic
- had a past stroke
- kidney disease
- diseased arteries elsewhere in the body (circulation problems)
- had one or more coronary bypass grafts already

The Disadvantages of Angioplasty

A Temporary Measure?

In general, angioplasty is very effective for treating symptoms of angina, and in selective cases, it may even extend life expectancy, but there is no evidence, at present, that it prevents heart attacks. Therefore, if you have an angioplasty you may still run the risk of your angina returning, or of suffering a heart attack in the future. No one is sure why this is, but it may have something to do with the fact that angioplasty does not remove the disease from all the blood vessel, which may cause problems in the future. By contrast, bypass surgery, which bypasses the entire diseased blood vessel, can prevent heart attacks *in some people* and extend life expectancy in the most severe forms of heart disease. These include people with severe disease of the left main artery, or disease of all three arteries *and* a weakened left ventricle, or diabetic people with disease in two or more blood vessels.

> "I loved the whole experience. I said, 'Can I watch the procedure?' and they said, 'Yes.' What I didn't enjoy was my recovery."
>
> **Arni Cohn**

This consideration may swing you in favor of bypass surgery, especially if you are young or have a young family, but bear in mind that this apparent advantage is based on studies done before recent advances in angioplasty technology, such as stents—now a routine part of most angioplasties. Because of this, it is difficult to truly compare current angioplasty procedures and bypass surgery. They may turn out to be equally effective. Recent studies suggest that bypass surgery and coronary angioplasty with stents have similar outcomes.

Risks of the Procedure

Angioplasty, like all medical procedures, carries a risk of complications—unwanted medical events that happen during or after the procedure. Some people are more at risk of complications than others and not all of the risks described below will apply to you. If you want some indication of your personal risks, talk to your physician.

The main risks of angioplasty and bypass surgery are shown in the More Detail box on page 46. Doctors divide risks into "early" complications (within hours or days) and "late" (long-term) complications.

The most frequent **early complication** is some bleeding or bruising at the incision site. Less common early complications are an aneurysm, where blood leaks out of the blood vessel at the site of the incision, or collapse of the coronary artery, due to the balloon

[MORE DETAIL]

*You **may** benefit more from bypass surgery than angioplasty if you have:*

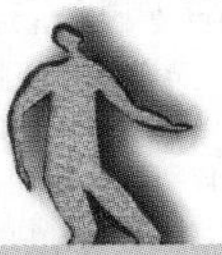

- a coronary artery that has been completely blocked for several weeks or months
- damaged heart valves or other condition that requires heart surgery
- coronary arteries narrowed in more than one place
- blockages in all three coronary arteries AND a weakened left ventricle (decreased heart muscle function)
- diabetes AND more than one blocked artery

tearing the artery wall during angioplasty. Sudden blockages in one or more coronary arteries can also occur during the procedure. This can lead to a small heart attack in 1 to 3 out of every 100 patients.

Another early complication is **perforation**, in which the wall of the coronary artery is pierced. This occurs in less than 1 in 1,000 simple angioplasties, but may lead to shock and immediate open-heart surgery. Not surprisingly, the risk of perforation increases as the procedure gets more complicated. The blood vessel innerwall may also be accidentally torn as the catheters are being inserted. This is called **dissection** and occurs in 20 to 40 percent of angioplasties. The problem can usually be fixed in the cath lab.

The most potentially serious early complication of angioplasty is a condition called **stent thrombosis**, where a blood clot forms on the metal stent, causing a blockage in the coronary artery and, thus, a heart attack. In the past, this complication occurred in up to 9 percent of patients after stent insertion. Nowadays, thanks to potent drugs that prevent blood clotting (see pages 50–51), and improved techniques of stent implantation, stent thrombosis occurs in less than 1 percent of people. Because of the potential for stent thrombosis, anti-platelet drugs must be continued for a minimum of 1 month after angioplasty to allow the blood vessel to cover the stent with the normal blood vessel lining.

In the long term, the most serious potential **late complication**

[MORE DETAIL]

Major Risks of Bypass Surgery

- Death in "low-risk" patients (1 to 3 percent)
- Heart attack (2 to 6 percent)
- Stroke (1 to 2 percent)
- Concentration and memory problems (estimates vary widely, from insignificant to one-quarter of patients at 6 months)
- Blood transfusion (10 percent or more)
- Return of angina (4 to 8 percent in the first year)

Major Risks of Angioplasty

- Death (0.5 to 1.4 percent)
- Heart attack (1 to 3 percent)
- Stroke (0.5 percent)
- Sudden blockage of coronary artery, resulting in emergency bypass surgery (0.2 to 3 percent)
- Blood transfusion (0.5 percent)
- Return of angina (15 to 30 percent with conventional stent)

of angioplasty is a condition called **re-stenosis**, where the coronary artery blocks up again several weeks or months later. This usually causes angina to return. This occurs in 30 to 40 percent of patients following balloon angioplasty alone, and 15 to 30 percent of patients who have had a conventional stent inserted. Newly available drug-coated stents appear to dramatically reduce the chances of re-stenosis (see pages 66–67).

For more on weighing up the risks of angioplasty, see pages 12–14, "Consent."

What Happens Next?

Unless your situation requires immediate treatment, it is reasonable to take as much time as you need to explore your options.

Although many people go ahead with their angioplasty right after their heart cath, others take the time to discuss things with family—or get a second medical opinion.

It is worth remembering, too, that angioplasty and bypass surgery can relieve your angina, but neither procedure actually cures your heart disease. Even if you have angioplasty or bypass surgery, you still need to make changes that will improve the health of your heart, otherwise your heart disease will continue to get worse. Take your medication correctly and don't forget to make lifestyle changes (see Chapter 11). Heart disease is a wake-up call: it's time to choose a different road.

"The doctor was always in a hurry; I wish he could have spent more time with me. I'd rather hear about the risks, then make up my own mind."

Robert (Bobby) Frew

Chapter 6

the angioplasty procedure

What Happens in this Chapter

- A step-by-step guide to your coronary angioplasty
- X-ray pictures during the procedure
- Use of blood-thinning drugs
- Insertion of the guide wire
- Balloon angioplasty
- Insertion of the stents
- Closing the incision

Coronary angioplasty, a procedure used to treat angina and heart attacks, was first performed in the late 1970s. It involves widening blocked coronary arteries by inflating a small balloon within the blocked region of the artery. Many sophisticated technologies have been added to this basic procedure over the years, including metal stents to keep the artery open, drills and cutters to remove blockages, and sophisticated blood-thinning drugs to improve patient safety. As a result of these improvements, angioplasty is now performed safely and effectively in the vast majority of patients, who can avoid bypass surgery and benefit from a quick recovery.

What is Coronary Angioplasty?

ANGIOPLASTY IS A TECHNIQUE USED TO WIDEN ANY ARTERY THAT has become blocked by fatty deposits in the artery walls. Coronary angioplasty is angioplasty of the coronary arteries—the crucial arteries that supply blood to the heart muscle. The procedure involves inserting a tube called a **guide catheter** into a major artery in the groin or wrist, then up to the heart and into the affected artery (see Figure 4–1). A thin wire (**guide wire**) is then passed down the guide catheter and across the blockage itself. A balloon is passed along the wire and inflated at the point of the obstruction (see Figure 6–1). This not only crushes the blockage against the sides of the artery, but also stretches the artery slightly, to widen it (see Figure 6–2). Often, a small metal tube called a **stent** is permanently placed in the artery to help keep the artery open (see Figure 6–4).

The technical term for this kind of procedure is **percutaneous coronary intervention (PCI)** because the guide wire and the balloon pass through a small incision in the skin ("percutaneous") to perform treatments, or medical "interventions."

The Angioplasty Equipment

Although you may not be aware of it during the procedure, angioplasty uses equipment that is slightly different from that used during your heart cath. First, the diameter of the catheters may be larger since some specialized and bulky angioplasty equipment requires extra-large catheters. Second, the guiding catheters are stiffer to provide extra support to the angioplasty equipment. As a result, it may take longer to insert the tip of the angioplasty guiding catheter into your narrowed blood vessel.

More Pictures

Your cardiologist will take more X-ray pictures throughout your angioplasty to guide him or her and to assess the results of the balloon inflation or stent insertion. Nitroglycerin, which you currently use to treat your angina attacks, may be injected directly down your narrowed coronary artery to help it relax before the pictures are taken.

Blood-Thinning Medication Before Your Procedure

Blood clotting is a natural process in which **platelets** (tiny cell fragments in the blood) and special blood proteins bind together to form a clot. It is a lifesaver at the right time and in the right place (for instance, after an injury), but is dangerous when it happens inside blood vessels. In this case, the blood clot could block the vessel and cut off blood flow, causing a heart attack. Blood clots are more likely to form when the blood flow meets an obstruction or makes contact with an injury on the artery wall. Both these situations are common during angioplasty, so you will need **blood-thinning medication** to ensure that all is well during the procedure.

To successfully prevent blood clotting—either in your blood vessels or on the angioplasty equipment—the activity of both the platelets and the blood-clotting proteins must be blocked.

You may already be taking ASA (Aspirin), a very common and inexpensive blood-thinner used by patients with coronary heart disease. ASA works by blocking the activity of platelets. For this reason, it is called an **anti-platelet drug**. Although ASA is effective in preventing most blood-clotting problems that happen after balloon angioplasty, it is less effective when a stent is used. Up to 1 percent of stents (tube-like supports placed inside coronary arteries) will block suddenly in the first week after angioplasty due to the formation of a blood clot inside the stent. To reduce the chances of this happening, additional anti-platelet drugs, such as **clopidogrel** (Plavix), will be given to you when you have an angioplasty with a stent. Clopidogrel, which works by further reducing the "stickiness" of platelets, is usually given to you before your procedure and taken for up to a year afterward. Recent studies have shown that, if taken for up to a year in combination with ASA (Aspirin), clopidogrel can reduce the risk of death, heart attacks, and strokes. If you are on another blood thinner, mention it to your medical team.

Blood-Thinning Medication During Your Angioplasty

Heparin

Heparin blocks the action of the blood-clotting proteins. It is given intravenously (into your vein) during your angioplasty and, in combination with your oral blood-thinning medication, such as ASA or clopidogrel, will significantly reduce your blood's ability to clot.

Special Blood Thinners

Recently, a new type of anti-platelet drug has been found to be useful in patients undergoing angioplasty. **Bivalirudin** (Angiomax) works in a similar way to heparin and is particularly helpful in treating heart attacks and unstable angina.

The **glycoprotein IIb/IIIa (or 2B-3A) inhibitors** act by blocking the clotting effects of platelets and are many times more powerful than oral blood thinners. They are only available for intravenous injection and are used during, and for up to 24 hours after, angioplasty.

These new, powerful anti-platelet drugs have been shown to be very effective in reducing the risk of a heart attack in patients undergoing angioplasty, with or without a stent, and even in some cases extending life expectancy. They can also reduce angina. They are often reserved for patients undergoing high-risk or difficult angioplasties, such as angioplasty during a heart attack. Overall, 60 to 80 percent of angioplasty patients in the United States receive them.

Your doctor will choose your blood-thinning medications based on your clinical condition, along with the findings during the heart catheterization.

To make sure that your blood is not over-thinned, a blood sample will be taken during your angioplasty for **activated clotting time (ACT)** and **partial thromboplastin time (PTT)** tests. The overall goal is to prevent blood clots, while, at the same time, making sure you do not suffer from bleeding complications. A balance is achieved in most cases, but bleeding or clotting complications do occur occasionally.

Insertion of the Guide Wire

The first important step during your angioplasty is "wiring the vessel." A long wire called a guide wire helps direct equipment such as balloons and stents into your narrowed blood vessel and through the actual narrowing (see Figure 6–1). The guide wire is first inserted into the guiding catheter and then, using the X-ray camera, its tip is carefully navigated down your blood vessel. You may see the guide wire moving down your blood vessel on the X-ray screen. Angioplasty guide wires are very small in diameter—only 14/1000 of an inch wide.

> "I think the fact that you can see what's happening on the television tends to keep your mind off things because you're watching what's going on, rather than just lying there and letting them do their thing.... And of course they have a bit of music going and the nurses are talking to you."
>
> **Bill Hogarth**

Figure 6–1. Keeping Angioplasty on Track

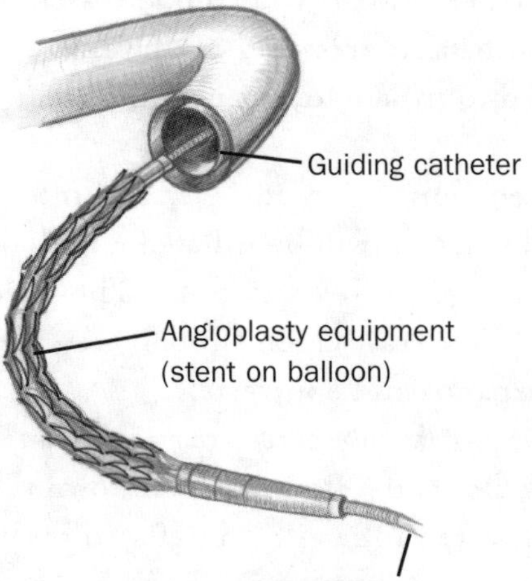

Just as a train runs on tracks through a subway tunnel, the angioplasty equipment travels to your heart on a guide wire through a guiding tube or catheter. The guide wire keeps the equipment on track as it moves into position at the site of blockage.

The insertion of a guide wire into a narrowed blood vessel rarely causes any problems, although it can sometimes cause angina symptoms. Occasionally, it is impossible for the physician to pass a guide wire through the narrowed region of a blood vessel. If this happens, it means, unfortunately, that your angioplasty cannot proceed because *all* angioplasty equipment needs a correctly positioned guide wire. This is more common if your blood vessel is totally blocked, rather than just narrowed, particularly if the complete blockage is more than a few months old.

Balloon Angioplasty

Once the guide wire is passed across the blockage, the next step is usually the use of an angioplasty balloon. Your cardiologist will insert the balloon along the guide wire and into your narrowed blood vessel. Angioplasty balloons were invented by a Swiss physician, Dr. Andreas Gruntzig, in the late 1970s. They are now available in a huge range of diameters and lengths, and your cardiologist will select one that exactly fits your blood vessel. These tough, plastic balloons can withstand pressures of up to 20 atmospheres and are designed to inflate to precisely the right diameter.

Once the balloon is inserted along the guide wire and into the narrowed area of your blood vessel, it will be inflated and deflated, using a hand-held pump (see Figures 6–2 and 6–3). The balloon is inflated with fluid visible on the X-ray screen (not air), so the physician can watch it as it expands and contracts.

Be forewarned: ***angina symptoms at this stage are very common*** because the inflated balloon temporarily blocks the flow of blood down the artery. Because the balloon is often inflated and deflated several times, you may feel angina pain coming and going. Your cardiologist should warn you each time you are likely to experience angina during your procedure. You will be kept comfortable and receive pain medication as needed throughout the procedure.

Figure 6–2. Balloon Angioplasty

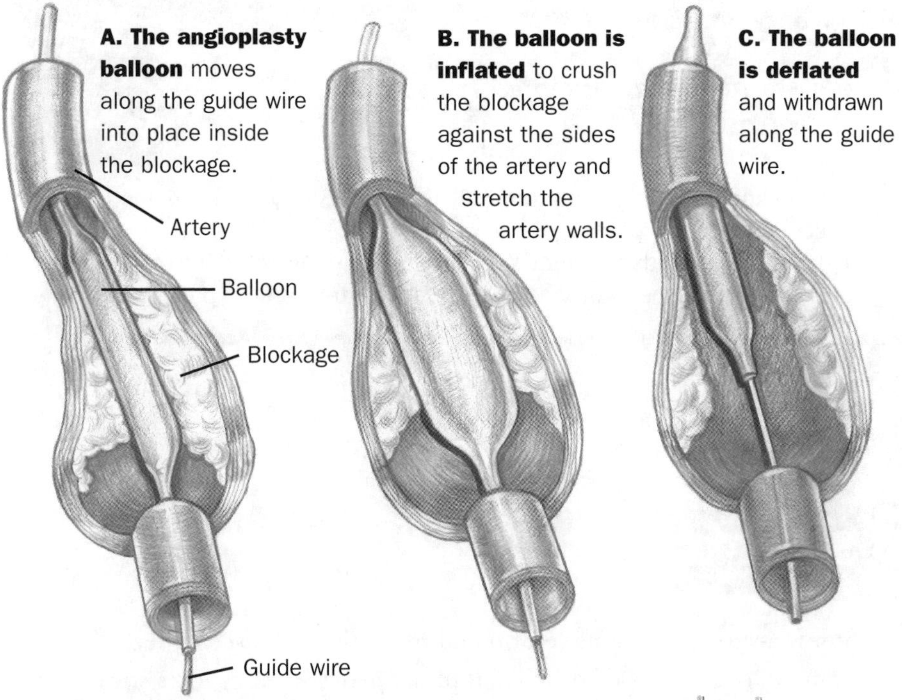
A. The angioplasty balloon moves along the guide wire into place inside the blockage.
Artery
Balloon
Blockage
Guide wire
B. The balloon is inflated to crush the blockage against the sides of the artery and stretch the artery walls.
C. The balloon is deflated and withdrawn along the guide wire.

Figure 6–3. Angioplasty Balloons

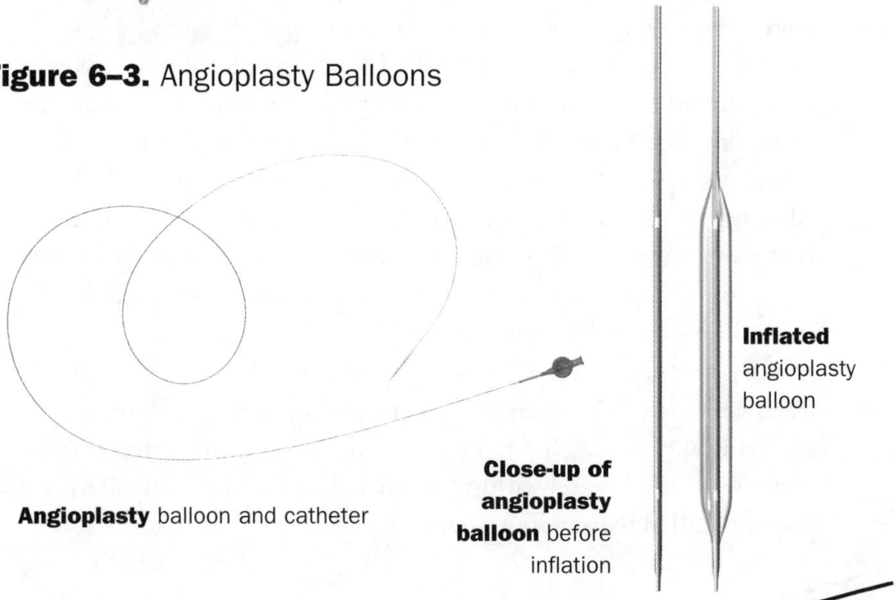
Angioplasty balloon and catheter
Close-up of angioplasty balloon before inflation
Inflated angioplasty balloon

[SELF-HELP]

Self-Help During Angioplasty

If you experience any symptoms AT ANY STAGE of your angioplasty procedure, inform your physician or nurse right away. You may experience a headache after the nitroglycerin is injected into the blood vessels. Do not be alarmed, you will feel better as time passes.

Stents

Stents are tiny tubes made of metal mesh that are used to try to improve the results of your angioplasty procedure. Studies show that angina returns in only 15 to 30 percent of patients who have stents inserted—up to half the rate for balloon angioplasty alone. New, drug-coated stents appear to improve results even more dramatically (see page 66). Stents have also significantly reduced the number of patients who need emergency bypass surgery after angioplasty. Although stenting does not provide perfect results, it is a definite improvement over balloon angioplasty alone. Whether you receive one or more stents depends on the size of your narrowed blood vessel and how long the narrowing is.

Early stents were relatively bulky and inflexible, so angioplasty physicians had to pre-stretch the narrowing with a balloon before inserting the stent. Modern stents can usually be inserted into a narrowed blood vessel without prior balloon angioplasty. This technique is called **direct stenting**.

A stent is usually delivered to the site of the blockage on an angioplasty balloon. As the balloon inflates, the stent enlarges and presses up against the sides of the blood vessel. Once the balloon is deflated and removed from the blood vessel, the stent is left behind to hold the walls of the blood vessel fully open (see Figures 6–4 and 6–5). Your physician may insert larger angioplasty balloons after your stent has been inserted to ensure full expansion of the stent—and a better long-term result. A small number of stents are self-expanding and do not require a balloon for insertion (although a balloon may be used to ensure that they are fully expanded) (see Figure 6–6).

Figure 6–4. Stent Insertion

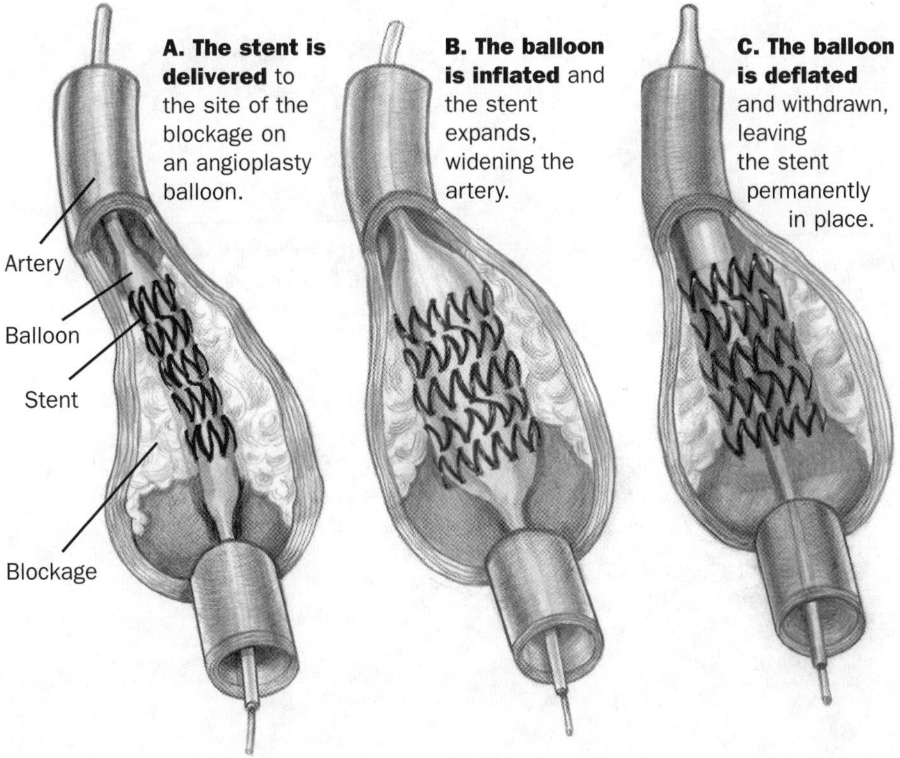
A. The stent is delivered to the site of the blockage on an angioplasty balloon.
B. The balloon is inflated and the stent expands, widening the artery.
C. The balloon is deflated and withdrawn, leaving the stent permanently in place.
Artery
Balloon
Stent
Blockage

Figure 6–5. Stents

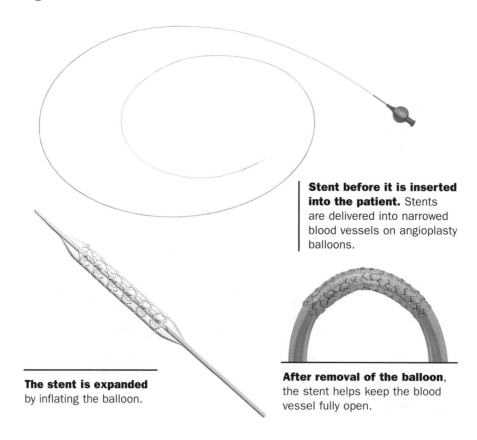

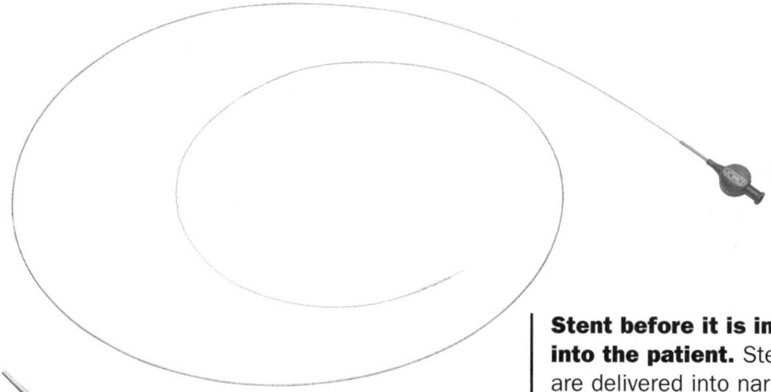

Stent before it is inserted into the patient. Stents are delivered into narrowed blood vessels on angioplasty balloons.

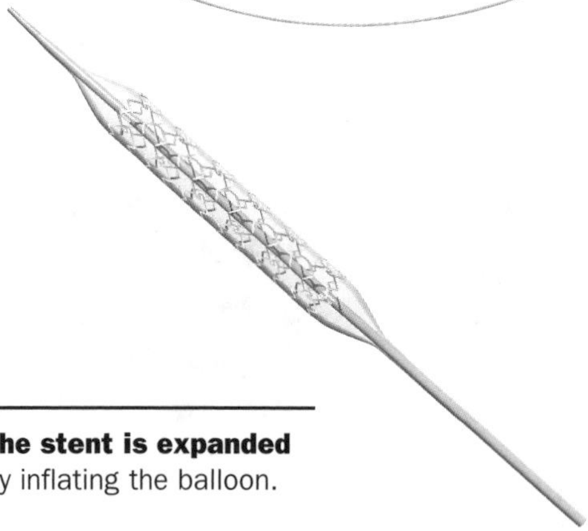

The stent is expanded by inflating the balloon.

After removal of the balloon, the stent helps keep the blood vessel fully open.

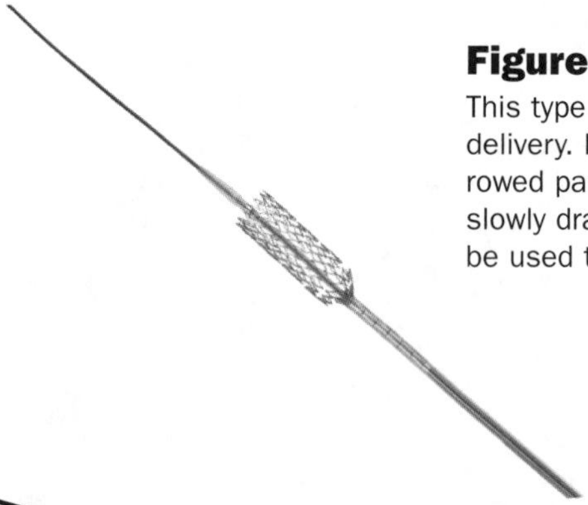

Figure 6–6. Self-Expanding Stent

This type of stent does not need a balloon for delivery. It expands automatically within the narrowed part of the artery as its outer covering is slowly drawn back. An angioplasty balloon may be used to complete the expansion.

Any symptoms that you may experience as a stent is put in place are similar to those of normal balloon angioplasty. You will not feel the stent being expanded or be aware of it afterward. In the following months, the artery wall will gradually grow over the stent and cover it completely.

"During the procedure they gave me a picture of before and after, of what the artery looked like before and what they did."

Mrs. C.V.

Although many different types of stents are available, there are few differences among them with respect to long-term results. On the whole, the long-term results of your angioplasty and stent will depend mainly on the size of your blood vessel and the length of the narrowed region. The type of stent that you will receive will depend upon which stent is available in your hospital and which stent your physician feels is most suitable for your blood vessel.

One of the downsides of stents is that they can suddenly block with a blood clot 3 to 5 days after angioplasty—a condition called stent thrombosis (see pages 45–46). Stents can also be difficult to unblock if they become narrowed in the future.

Other Angioplasty Techniques

Apart from balloons and stents, there is an increasing number of sophisticated angioplasty tools and techniques that your physician can use to help you. These are covered in Chapter 7, along with their advantages and disadvantages.

Closing the Incision

Because of all the blood-thinning medication you were given, you are at a higher risk of bleeding immediately after your angioplasty than after your heart cath alone. What happens next will depend on whether your wrist or groin was used and whether your physician uses a closure device.

Conventional Approach—Late Sheath Removal

If you have had angioplasty via your groin, the standard approach is to leave the sheath in place for 4 to 6 hours after your angioplasty, during which time you will be lying flat on your back in the recovery area (see page 79). This allows time for some of your blood-thinning medication to wear off.

> "They explained about pressure and the fact they had cut into a major artery and they had to seal the wound. The clamp looked like a huge vise, with one part underneath the mattress for stability. I was stuck in this big thing and thinking, 'I wonder who thought of this?'"
>
> **Arni Cohn**

Closure Devices—Immediate Sheath Removal

One of the alternatives to late sheath removal is the use of closure devices, which can halve the time you need to spend in bed. There are a number of different designs, but they all work basically the same way—by either plugging or tying shut the hole in your leg artery. Closure devices need to be put on in a sterile environment, so they are applied in the cath lab at the end of your angioplasty procedure. This usually adds only a few minutes to the end of your procedure. Closure devices allow you to move around a few hours after your angioplasty and, potentially, allow safe, early discharge from the hospital. Complications are uncommon with closure devices, but they do happen occasionally. These include damage to the artery or failure to prevent bleeding (in which case manual pressure may be used).

At the End of Your Angioplasty

At the end of your angioplasty procedure, you should expect to be free of pain. If this is not the case, tell your cardiologist. Very occasionally, an angioplasty patient may experience chest discomfort for a few hours after the procedure—for instance, due to blockage of a small side branch of the vessel caused by the balloon or stent. It is not always possible to keep all small side branches open when performing angioplasty. If this type of blockage occurs, it should be visible on your final X-ray pictures and your cardiologist may prescribe pain-relieving medication. The pain should subside after a few hours. Very occasionally, this situation can result in a small heart attack. If this happens, it will be confirmed by blood tests taken the day after your angioplasty.

What Happens Next?

After your angioplasty is completed, you will be transferred to a special ward or recovery area. Here, you will learn how to care for your wound and how to take care of yourself while you are healing. Chapter 9 lets you know what will happen immediately after your procedure.

Chapter 7

the angioplasty toolkit

What Happens in this Chapter

- A more detailed look at the tools your physician may use in the angioplasty procedure
- The low-down on drug-coated stents, atherectomy, thrombectomy, lasers, brachytherapy and distal protection devices
- Other techniques your physician may use to help you

There are a number of ways to improve the blood flow down your narrowed or blocked arteries. Some are better than others in terms of their short- and long-term results and some are more suitable for certain kinds of narrowings than others. While you will not be able to choose the tools that your physician selects, knowing something about the angioplasty toolkit may help you feel more in control of your procedure.

Opening up the Toolkit

In Chapters 4 and 6 we looked at the basic steps of your heart cath and angioplasty. You may feel that this is all you need (or want) to know about your procedures. However, if you want more detail on the sophisticated tools and techniques that your physician may use, this is the chapter for you.

Atherectomy Devices

Neither balloon angioplasty nor stent insertion removes any of the brittle, fatty blockage (**atherosclerotic plaque**) from the walls of narrowed blood vessels. For this, cutting devices called **atherectomy devices** are needed. Removing some of the plaque before balloon angioplasty or stent insertion can make it easier for the physician to inflate the balloon or open the stent completely.

A disadvantage of atherectomy devices in general is that they need large guiding catheters that may be more uncomfortable for the patient. There is also a slightly increased risk of complications, such as heart attack, in part because atherectomy is traditionally used to treat complex blockages.

Directional atherectomy devices incorporate a cutting blade and balloon into the end of a catheter. They may prove to be particularly useful in patients with a severe blockage on just one side of the blood vessel wall or whose stents have become blocked. The latest devices, such as the one in Figure 7–1, may be particularly helpful for patients with a lot of calcium in their artery walls.

Rotational atherectomy devices are drill-like devices for removing plaque (see Figure 7–2). Rotational atherectomy may be particularly useful for removing large quantities of plaque and very long or very hard blockages.

If you are having rotational atherectomy, you may need a temporary pacemaker inserted before your angioplasty.

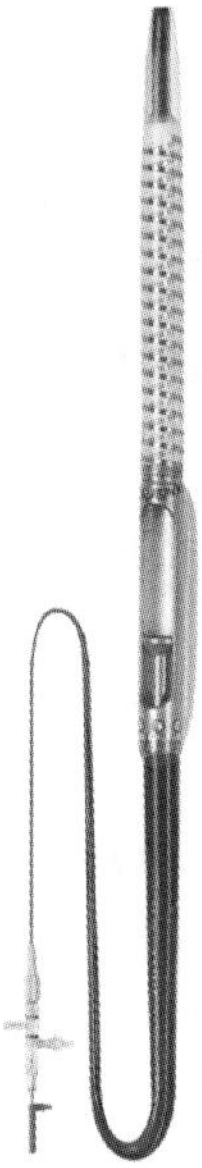

Figure 7–1. Directional Atherectomy Device **This combined balloon and cutter**, called the FLEXI-CUT™ Directional Debulking System, slices plaque off the blood vessel wall. The debris is then collected and removed by the catheter.

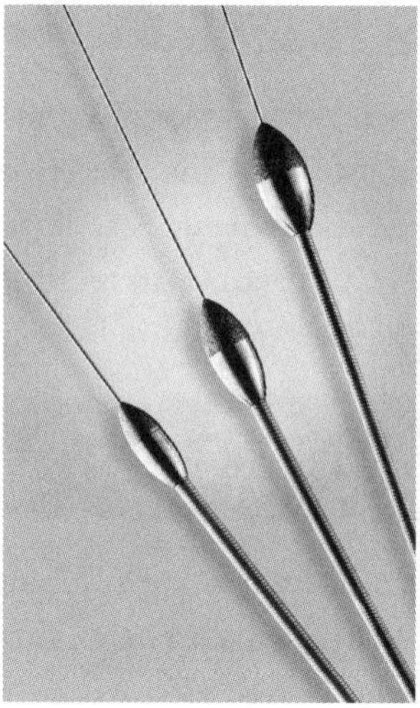

Figure 7–2. Rotational Atherectomy Device **This diamond-encrusted, olive-shaped device**, called the Rotablator® Rotational Atherectomy System, rotates at high speed to remove hard, calcified blockages.

Thrombectomy Devices

A blood clot (**thrombus**) is common in coronary arteries of patients with severe or recent angina, or those who are having a heart attack (see Figure 1–1, page 3). Sometimes a thrombus can form during the angioplasty procedure itself, increasing the risk of a heart attack and other long- and short-term complications. To reduce this risk, your physician may use a **thrombectomy device** before he or she inserts an angioplasty balloon and stent. Currently, these devices effectively remove blood clots by suction (see Figure 7–3), although their long-term benefits have yet to be proven in clinical studies. Thrombectomy may be more uncomfortable than balloon angioplasty because larger guiding catheters are used.

Figure 7–3. Thrombectomy Device

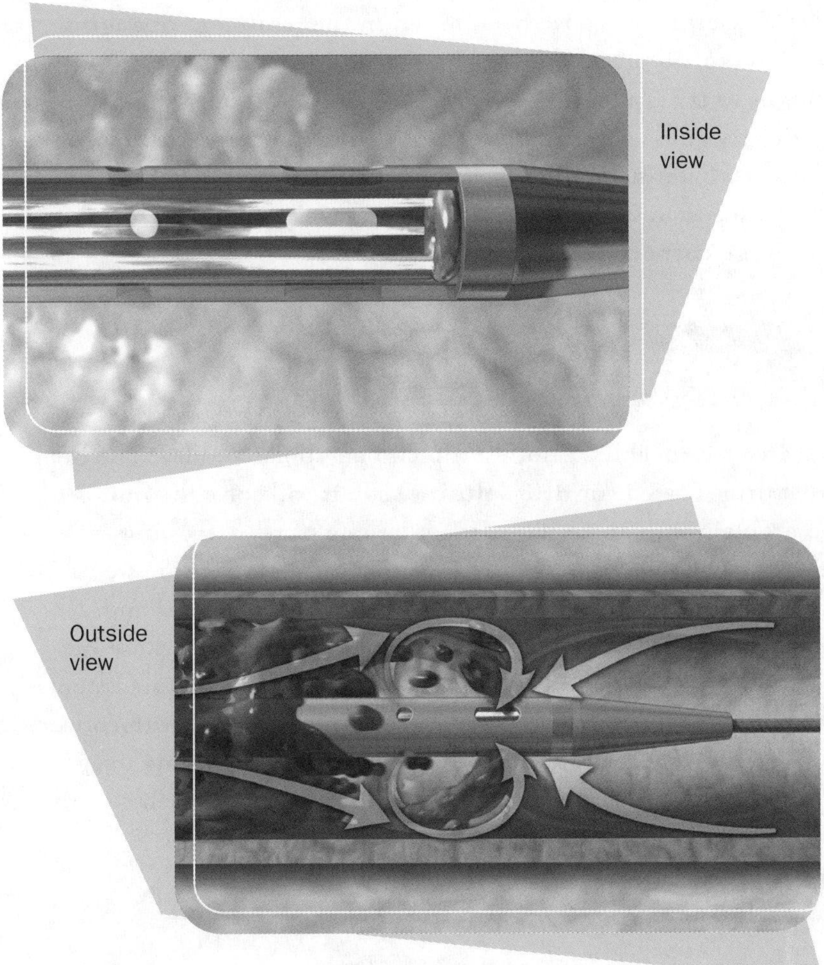

The AngioJet® Rheolytic™ Thrombectomy System works by suctioning blood clots into the catheter and breaking them up with saline jets that travel at half the speed of sound.

Laser Devices

Various laser devices have been tested in the treatment of angina with little or no success. Lasers have been incorporated into balloons to try to improve angioplasty results and onto the tips of angioplasty guide wires to help them pass through blocked blood vessels. To date, no studies have demonstrated the advantages of any laser device in any situation. Most laser devices are now gathering dust in the corners of cath labs.

Drug-Coated Stents

This area is probably *the* hottest topic in angioplasty today. The hope is that drug-coated (or **drug-eluting**) stents will solve the number one problem with angioplasty: the high rate of re-narrowing (re-stenosis). Their aim is to reduce scar formation inside stents, which reduces the open space in the blood vessel (**lumen**) and the flow of blood. Side effects for the patient are unlikely because the drug only goes to where it is needed. In general, drug-coated stents have reduced re-blockage by over 50 percent compared with conventional stents. There are now several companies developing drug-eluting stents and some of these stents will become available in the

Figure 7–4. Drug-Coated Stent

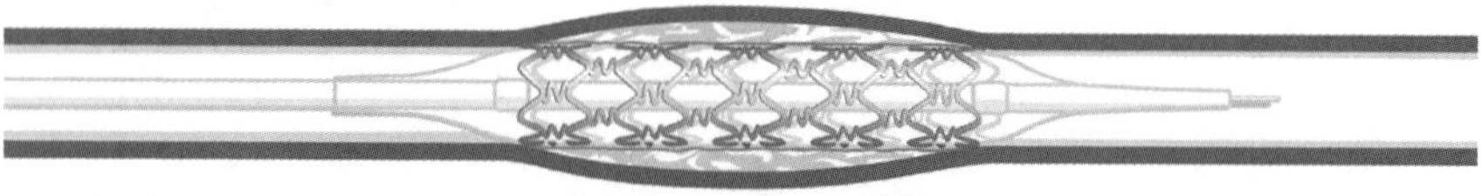

This drug-coated stent, called the CYPHER™ Sirolimus-Eluting Stent, significantly reduces artery re-narrowing. It is a new device that is on the cutting edge of stent technology.

United States in 2003. These stents are more expensive than regular stents and researchers are still trying to find out which type of patient will benefit most from them.

Brachytherapy

Brachytherapy is a way of using radiation to try to prevent re-narrowing after angioplasty (see Figure 7–5). It may prove to be the best way to deal with stents that have re-narrowed along their entire lengths. However, there is no evidence so far that brachytherapy prevents re-narrowing in arteries *without stents*. It also means additional exposure to radiation and a longer, more complicated procedure that requires the combined skills of a cardiologist and a radiation oncologist (cancer specialist).

There are two types of brachytherapy: one uses **gamma radiation** and the other uses **beta radiation**. Gamma radiation is more powerful than beta, but it requires special radiation shielding in the cath labs. Therefore, beta radiation is the most commonly used system in the United States. The radiation is turned on for typically 20 to 30 seconds.

Figure 7–5. Brachytherapy Device

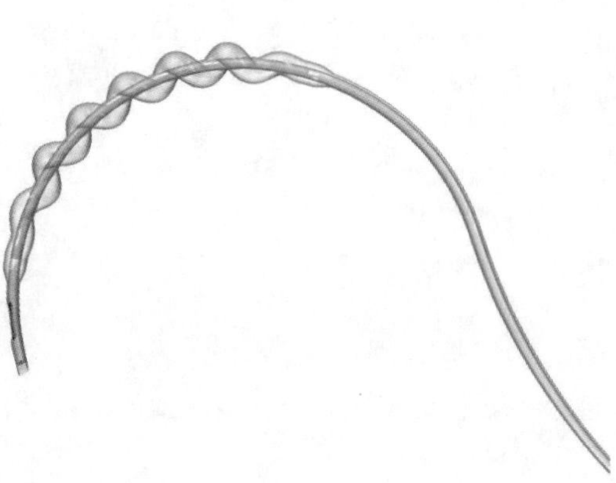

This spiral-like balloon, called the GALILEO™ Centering Catheter, uses radiation to reduce the re-narrowing of stents. The radioactive material is on the tip of a wire that is inserted into the center of the balloon. The spiral balloon may allow blood to flow down the artery while applying radiation equally throughout the artery's length and width.

Cutting Balloon™ Device

The **Cutting Balloon device** is similar to an ordinary angioplasty balloon, but it allows the blockage to be pushed against the artery wall more easily (see Figure 7–6). This means that it can open blockages with much lower pressure than a conventional balloon and, therefore, reduces the injury to the artery wall. Some studies show that it also reduces the rate of re-narrowing. Cutting Balloon devices may prove to be especially beneficial for blockages at the entrance of a blood vessel or inside a stent, and in vein grafts after bypass surgery.

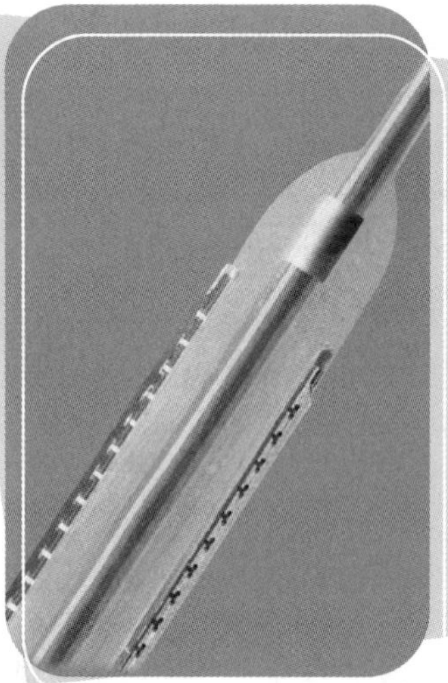

Figure 7–6
Cutting Balloon™ Device
This angioplasty balloon has three or four blades attached to the outside that cut into the hard blockage when the balloon is inflated. This makes the artery wall less rigid and easier to stretch.

Distal Protection Devices

In some types of blood vessels and blockages, when the angioplasty balloon inflates, pieces of plaque fall off and get carried downstream, where they block smaller arteries. This is called **distal embolization**, and can result in a slowing or stopping of the heartbeat, angina, or even a heart attack.

Distal embolization is more common in angioplasty of bypass grafts and where the narrowed part of the artery contains a blood clot. To prevent distal embolization in these types of narrowings, specially designed catheters can be used to catch the debris before it gets swept away. Several different types of devices are currently under development (see Figure 7–7).

Although for technical reasons they can't be used every time, these devices have proved to be excellent. They are particularly useful for patients undergoing angioplasty or stent placement in bypass grafts, where quite a bit of debris can get into the circulation. Over time, these devices are likely to be used more routinely in certain types of "high-risk" patient.

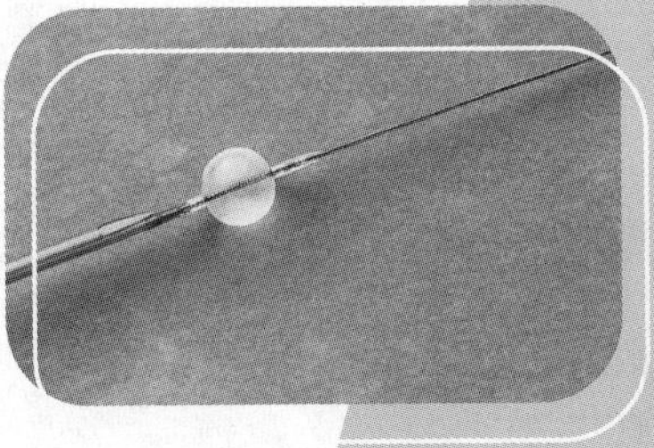

Figure 7–7.
PercuSurge™ Device
The special balloon is positioned beyond the blockage before the angioplasty balloon is inflated. Any debris that falls from the artery wall is trapped within the vessel, since there is no flow, and removed by the suction tube.

Additional (Adjunctive) Techniques and Devices

In addition to the techniques available to treat narrowed or blocked blood vessels, several devices can be used to help improve their long-term results.

Intravascular Ultrasound

The use of **ultrasound** in general (using sound waves bounced off part of the body to form an image) has had a huge impact in all fields of medicine. It is used to diagnose disease, to check the health of an unborn baby, and as a treatment. You may have had a cardiac ultrasound to assess the strength of your heart muscle or the function of your heart valves.

An ultrasound probe (which sends and receives sound waves to build up a picture of your heart) can now be miniaturized and inserted into blood vessels in a procedure called **intravascular ultrasound** (**IVUS**). This is normally performed as part of an angioplasty, or is occasionally done during an angiogram. It provides more accurate images of your blood vessels than angiography does (see Figure 7–8). A recent study has shown that arteries are less likely to re-narrow if IVUS is used to guide the placement of a stent. IVUS is not a routine procedure in the U.S., but it is useful for some kinds of angioplasties.

Figure 7–8. The inside of a coronary artery, as revealed by IVUS (intravascular ultrasound)

IVUS provides a more accurate picture of an artery, including the central space (the lumen), the wall, and any blockages (plaque). By comparison, a coronary angiogram only reveals the lumen.

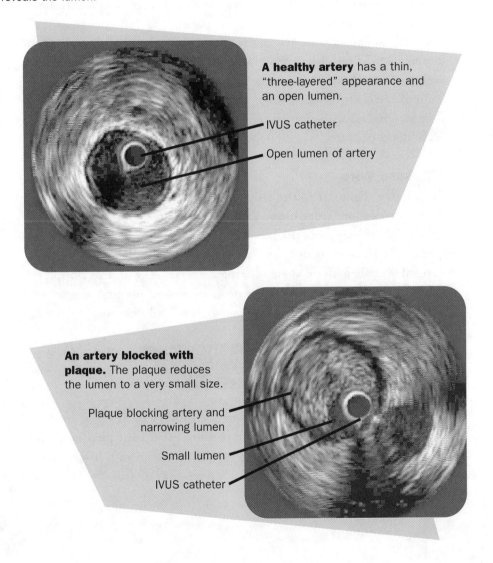

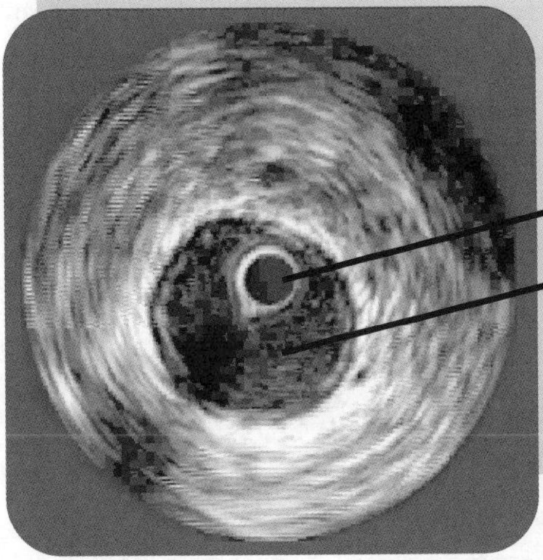

A healthy artery has a thin, "three-layered" appearance and an open lumen.

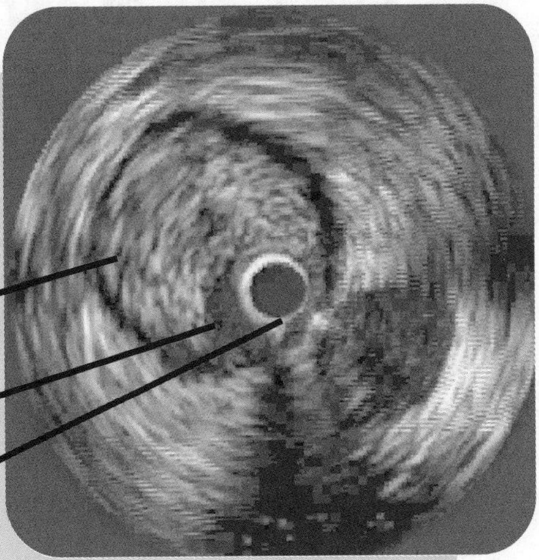

An artery blocked with plaque. The plaque reduces the lumen to a very small size.

Doppler Flow Wire

A **Doppler flow wire** uses ultrasound to measure the actual blood flow down coronary arteries in the same way that radar guns are used by traffic police to measure the speed of vehicles. The ultrasound device is mounted onto the end of a very small wire, similar to the angioplasty guide wire.

Blood flow in healthy arteries increases by a factor of three during exercise. In the cath lab, a short-acting drug is usually given to simulate exercise. The Doppler flow wire is then used to decide whether an angioplasty is required or when it has been successful. The Doppler flow wire may not give accurate results for people with diabetes or high blood pressure.

Pressure Wire

This device is similar to the Doppler flow wire, but instead of using sound waves to measure blood flow, the **pressure wire** measures the drop in pressure across the blockage. In normal or mildly narrowed blood vessels, there is only a small drop in pressure (less than 25 percent) inside a blood vessel during exercise. As with the Doppler flow wire, a drug is used to simulate exercise and the pressure wire then measures the degree of blockage before and after angioplasty.

What Happens Next?

Everyone is different, and cardiology technology moves fast, so if you have any questions about the techniques that your physician may use in your particular case, be sure to discuss them with him or her before your procedure.

Chapter 8

angioplasty in other parts of the body

What Happens in this Chapter

- Why you might need peripheral angioplasty
- The peripheral angioplasty procedure
- Risks of different peripheral angioplasties

The aim of performing peripheral angioplasty, or angioplasty in blood vessels outside the heart, is identical to that of the coronary arteries: namely, to stretch narrowed arteries, allowing blood to flow freely once more. The basic techniques involved for different kinds of angioplasties are also similar. The main differences between coronary and peripheral angioplasty include treatment goals, the size of the arteries involved, and the complications that you may experience.

What is Peripheral Angioplasty?

PERIPHERAL ANGIOPLASTY (**PERIPHERAL TRANSLUMINAL angioplasty**, or **PTA**) is a procedure that widens blocked arteries in parts of the body other than the heart. Angioplasty is often thought of as a heart operation, but it can be very effective in organs such as lower limbs, kidneys, stomach and intestines, aorta, and head and neck.

Coronary Angioplasty vs. Peripheral Angioplasty

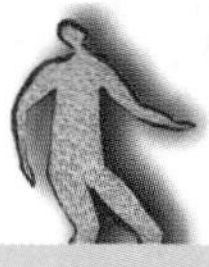

[MORE DETAIL]

The following are the main differences between angioplasty in the heart and angioplasty in other parts of the body:

- **Reasons for treatment.** In the heart, angioplasty relieves angina; in the kidney, it reduces blood pressure; in the legs, it reduces walking pain (**claudication**).
- **Sizes of arteries.** Outside the heart, the size range of arteries varies widely. This may explain why some peripheral arteries can be treated with balloons alone, and others need stents.
- **Different risks.** Stroke is more common during angioplasty of the head and neck arteries, for instance, than during coronary angioplasty.

Figure 8–1. Peripheral Angioplasty

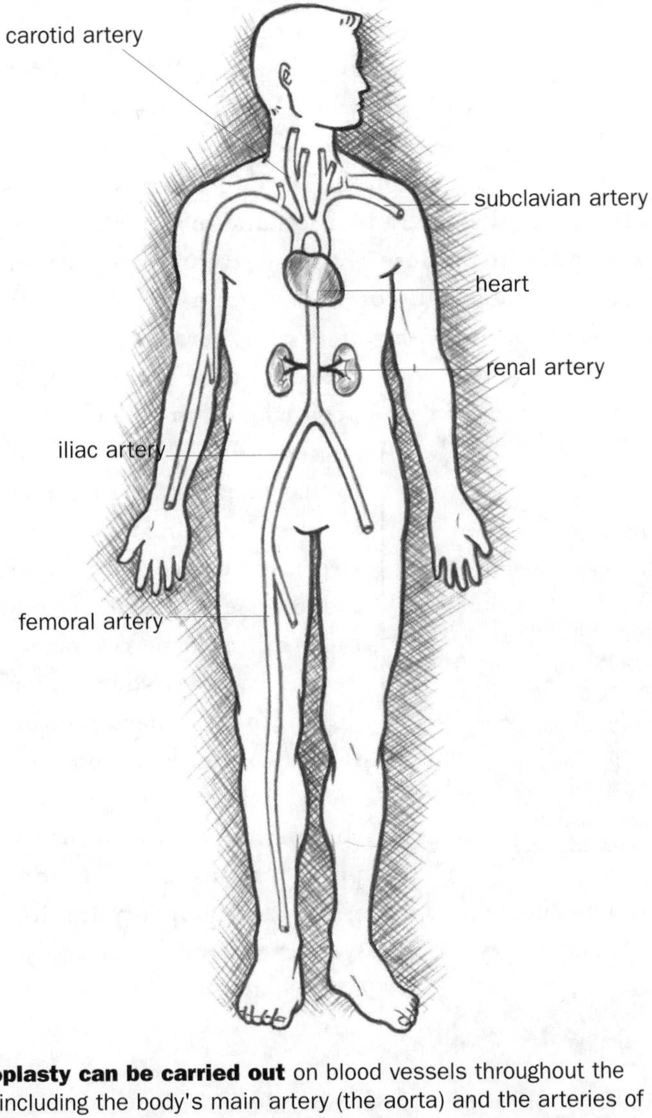

Angioplasty can be carried out on blood vessels throughout the body, including the body's main artery (the aorta) and the arteries of the legs, stomach, kidneys, and neck. As for coronary angioplasty, the point of entry for peripheral angioplasty is a blood vessel in the arm or leg.

Your Procedure

Your cardiologist may perform angiography of non-coronary arteries at the same time as your heart cath if he or she thinks that you might have **peripheral vascular disease (PVD)**, or blockages in your lower limbs, kidneys, stomach and intestines, aorta, or head and neck vessels. The angiography of vessels in other parts of your body is performed through the same incision as your heart cath, so you will not need an extra incision and may not realize that pictures of vessels other than those of your heart are being taken.

If your cardiologist discovers that you have PVD, he or she will discuss your options with you. If peripheral angioplasty is recommended and you give your consent for the procedure, it is usually performed immediately after your angiography. The procedure is similar to that of coronary angioplasty in that it involves inserting a balloon, or other stretching device, into the blocked blood vessel through a small incision in the groin or arm. You may require a new incision for your angioplasty, depending on where your blockages are. If you wish to think about your treatment decision after your angiography, you may ask your cardiologist to end the procedure instead of performing angioplasty. The alternatives to peripheral angioplasty are the same as those for coronary angioplasty—drug therapy or surgery.

[KEY POINT]

The preparation, procedures, equipment, drugs, consent, and self-help for peripheral angioplasty are similar to those for coronary angioplasty, so don't forget to check out the rest of the book for more on these topics.

Risks

Possible complications of peripheral angioplasty include bleeding and bruising from the place where your sheath is inserted, rupture or blockage of the narrowed artery, and, in the long-term, re-narrowing of the blood vessel (re-stenosis). As well as the general risks that apply to all peripheral angioplasties, the main risks of angioplasty of the kidneys are that your kidney function may actually get worse and, immediately after your procedure, your blood pressure may fall too low. The most significant risk of carotid angioplasty is having a stroke or a "mini-stroke" during, or shortly after, the procedure. This occurs in 3 percent of cases and is caused by pieces of the fatty blockage breaking off during balloon inflation and lodging in the blood vessels of the brain (distal embolization). Other potential complications of carotid angioplasty include slowing of the heart rate and a lowering of blood pressure.

Did It Work?

Your peripheral angioplasty will be considered a success if your blood vessel remains open in the long-term. In your legs this will mean that you can walk for longer distances because your symptoms of leg cramping are resolved or greatly reduced. In severe disease, the threat of amputation should be averted. If you had renal angioplasty, you will be hoping for improvements in your kidney function and blood pressure.

What Happens Next?

After your procedure you will be transferred to a recovery area or ward, where you will be kept under close observation by a nurse to ensure that no complications develop, either at your angioplasty site or at the point of the incision in your groin or arm. If no complications develop overnight, you will be allowed to go home the next day.

Chapter 9

when it's all over

What Happens in this Chapter

- The immediate aftermath
- Your return to the ward
- Symptoms to watch for
- Care of your wound
- Eating and drinking
- Going home checklist

The recovery from a heart cath alone is similar to the recovery from angioplasty. You will need to stay in bed, lying flat while your puncture closes. Nursing staff will keep an eye on you to check that all is well. If you had only a heart cath, you will be allowed to go home a few hours after your procedure. If you had an angioplasty, you will remain in the hospital for observation overnight and then sent home the next day unless a complication has occurred.

After Your Heart Cath

ONCE YOUR HEART CATH IS OVER AND YOU DO NOT NEED FURTHER treatment in the cath lab, the sheath in your groin through which the catheters were inserted will usually be removed immediately. To form a blood clot and reduce the risk of bleeding from the wound until the artery heals, a cath lab team member will either apply pressure manually (by pressing on your arm or groin with his or her hands) or use a specially designed clamp-like device. Pressure, however applied, is usually needed for up to 30 minutes. You will be kept in bed for a few hours before being allowed to walk around to make sure that the blood vessel does not start to bleed again. During this period, you and your puncture site will be closely supervised by a nurse. In some hospitals, your blood vessel will have been sealed using a special piece of equipment called a **closure device** (see pages 60-61). If there are no complications during your recovery, you will be allowed to go home that same day.

After Your Angioplasty

As soon as your angioplasty has finished, you will be transferred—still flat on your back—to a recovery area or directly back to the ward. If you have had your angioplasty via your groin, you will not be allowed to sit up for several hours. You may find this uncomfortable and difficult to tolerate, particularly if your angioplasty procedure took a long time, but there are some good reasons for it. The amount of sedative and the effect it has varies from patient to patient, but the medical and nursing staff will want to make sure that you are no longer groggy before you get out of bed. There is also a risk of bleeding or bruising if you sit up in bed or get out of bed too early since angioplasty involves a puncture in a major artery. Moreover, your blood is "thinner" from the blood-thinning drugs needed for your angioplasty.

Arrival Back on the Ward

After your angioplasty your medical team will do everything they can to ensure that you have a safe recovery. To prevent problems from arising, or to ensure that any problems are dealt with quickly, the nursing staff will take a number of precautions upon your arrival in the ward or recovery area:

> "They gave me painkillers when we left the operating room because I asked. Whatever I wanted in terms of pain relief, they gave me."
>
> **Arni Cohn**

- The nurse accompanying you from the cath lab will give a short report to the ward or recovery-area nurse. This will normally include a brief summary of your procedure, the drugs given to you in the cath lab, additional drugs that may be needed after your procedure, and any problems that occurred during your angioplasty. He or she will also mention specific problems for your nurse to watch for.

- You will be asked if you have any symptoms such as chest discomfort or breathlessness. Don't try to be "brave." If you have any symptoms, mention them right away.

- The site of the puncture will be checked regularly for signs of bleeding or bruising because your blood will be thin for the first few hours after your angioplasty.
- A blood sample will be taken for routine testing.
- You will be connected to a heart monitor that displays your heart rhythms at all times.
- A routine ECG will be performed.
- Your "vital signs" (heart rate and blood pressure) will be checked regularly. This may involve the use of an automatic blood pressure machine pre-set to measure your blood pressure every few minutes after you arrive on the ward. Blood pressure and heart-rate checks will become less frequent as time goes on.
- Your intravenous lines will be checked to ensure that they are running properly and that the correct dose is being delivered to you.

Friends and Family

After your angioplasty, friends and family will no doubt be anxious to know how you are and to hear about what happened. You may also be keen to speak to them. However, your safety comes first. Before you have visitors, the nursing and medical staff need to check your condition and carry out the safety procedures listed above. Once these have been performed and your condition has been confirmed as stable and satisfactory, your family will be allowed to see you.

What If I Get Chest Discomfort?

You may experience slight chest pain or discomfort at the end of your angioplasty. Your physician will try to prevent this or treat it while you are in the cath lab, but this may not be possible, in which case you will leave the cath lab with some leftover chest discomfort. This usually improves gradually over the next few minutes or hours.

The most likely reason for discomfort after an otherwise successful angioplasty is angina due to blockage of one or more of the tiny blood vessels that branch off the main blood vessel dilated by the balloon. If your medical team identifies this as the cause of your lingering chest pain, they will give you a pain-relieving injection. You should still tell your nurse if the discomfort gets worse or does not improve over time. Remember, too, that angina can be experienced as arm, neck, or back discomfort or tightness—not just chest pain. Be sure to mention any upper-body symptoms to your nurse.

[KEY POINT]

If you get any chest discomfort at any time after your angioplasty, inform your nurse immediately.

If you have no pain when you leave the cath lab, but start to develop discomfort afterward, your medical team will check you over carefully before you are given pain medication. Your heart rate and blood pressure will be measured and, possibly, a new ECG taken. What happens next will depend on what the tests show. If your chest discomfort continues, you may simply be given nitroglycerine under your tongue or a strong pain-relieving drug such as morphine. In the unlikely event that your chest pain is due to re-narrowing or blockage of your blood vessel, you will need to be taken back to the cath lab for a repeat heart cath and, possibly, a further angioplasty.

Blood Tests

Blood tests will be done routinely after your angioplasty.

Very infrequently, the number of platelets in the blood (**blood count**) can fall as a side effect of all the blood-thinning drugs and injections involved in the angioplasty procedure. Having an adequate blood count is important because platelets help blood to clot. If your blood count does fall, you will be at risk of bleeding from your groin until the wound fully heals. As a matter of routine, your blood count will also be re-checked the day after your procedure and before you are discharged from the hospital.

> "I can remember my body tilting when they put the pressure on the one side. It's very uncomfortable and there's a certain amount of indignity when you have to go to the bathroom, but that's to be expected...it's like having your tooth out and saying, 'Well, I've got to eat soup the next couple of days.' It just kind-of goes with the procedure. And after the one day—you're done."
>
> **Bill Hogarth**

Your blood will also be tested to check for damage to your heart. Sensitive blood tests are now available, called **troponin tests**, that can detect even the slightest damage. Using such tests, recent studies have shown that some people suffer very small heart attacks during or after angioplasty that would otherwise go undetected. Although physicians are still debating whether these very small heart attacks are significant, if your troponin test comes out positive you may need to stay in the hospital a little longer and have some further tests as a precaution.

Your kidney function will be evaluated through blood tests, as well. This is done to make sure that the dye has not harmed your kidneys.

Care of Your Wound

Once you return to the ward, the nursing staff will check the site of your puncture or wound frequently. You should also be aware of how you feel and keep a look out for symptoms such as bleeding, swelling, or pain. Let your nurse know immediately if anything is bothering you. What happens next with your puncture depends on how your angioplasty was performed.

Late Sheath Removal

If your angioplasty was performed via your groin, your physician may leave the sheath in place for a few hours after your procedure, held in place by a small stitch (**suture**) or tie. This is the traditional approach and is done to allow the effect of the blood-thinning drugs to wear off a bit before your sheath is removed to reduce the chances of bleeding or bruising. It also allows a repeat angioplasty to be performed quickly if the blood vessel re-narrows or blocks any time after your procedure.

If the sheath is left in place, you will be kept flat on your back in bed for 4 to 6 hours before it can be removed. *You will not be able to bend your leg—even for a moment—because the sheath will bend inside the artery and cut off the blood supply to your leg.*

The exact amount of time the sheath stays in your groin can vary from hospital to hospital. It can also depend on the results of your blood tests. Once your sheath is removed, you will have to stay in bed for a further 4 to 6 hours, still lying completely flat. Your nurse may place a sandbag or clamp on your groin to provide extra pressure. Overall, with this method, you will be in bed for about 10 to 12 hours, and occasionally longer.

To remove your sheath, your medical team will give you a local anesthetic injection and then snip the suture holding the sheath in place. The sheath will then be pulled from your groin and a clamp or manual pressure will be applied to the area for 15 to 30 minutes to prevent bleeding. Sheath removal may be a little uncomfortable, but is not usually painful.

Once the sheath is out and there is no sign of bleeding, the manual pressure will be released or the clamp removed. Nursing staff will continue to keep an eye on you in case of further bleeding.

Closure Devices for Your Groin

One of the alternatives to prolonged bed rest is the use of closure devices, (see pages 60-61), which can halve the time you need to spend in bed. If you have a closure device, you may be allowed out of bed after 4 to 6 hours, although you will need to lie flat for much of this time. As with a sheath, your closure device will be checked at regular intervals and, if you become aware of any bleeding, you should let your nurse know.

> "The sheath came out sometime in the afternoon, although I can't remember it very well. There is no pain, the only discomfort is afterwards, when you can't move."
>
> Mrs. C.V.

Angioplasty Via Your Wrist

If your angioplasty has been performed via your wrist, the sheath is removed immediately and replaced by a small clamp or tight bandage to stop any bleeding. When this has been done, you can sit up in bed right away. You may even be transferred to your ward in a wheelchair rather than a bed. There is some bed rest, but much less than with groin angioplasty, and you will be able to get out of bed within a few hours.

Once back on the ward after your wrist angioplasty, your nurse will check your wrist at regular intervals for bruising, swelling, or bleeding. The bandage or clamp on your wrist is normally removed after 1 to 2 hours and replaced with a small adhesive bandage.

Eating and Drinking

There are two main limitations to eating and drinking after angioplasty. First, it is difficult to eat and drink while you are lying flat in bed. Second, food and drink are normally delayed for a few hours after your angioplasty as a precaution in case any complications develop. In the unlikely event that your blood vessel did re-narrow or block in the first few hours after your angioplasty, you may need to have another angioplasty or, possibly, an emergency bypass operation. Some hospitals like to wait until your sheath is removed before letting you eat or drink. So even though you will be hungry, you will still need to wait a few hours after your angioplasty before eating and drinking. Once this precautionary period is over, you should be able to eat and drink normally. However, all hospitals have different policies regarding eating after angioplasty.

> "It's strange when you're on your back and they bring you lunch... eating sandwiches lying down isn't easy."
>
> **Bill Hogarth**

Discharge

The number of days that patients spend in the hospital after an angioplasty has fallen over the years because angioplasty techniques have improved. You will probably only spend one night in the hospital after your angioplasty before being discharged, although this will depend on the severity of your heart problems and how well you recover from the angioplasty. Some hospitals in Europe are starting to send patients with successful angioplasties home later the same day and angioplasty is viewed as just another day surgery or minor surgical procedure. This is still uncommon in the U.S. and, in general, not recommended by the American College of Cardiology.

Pre-Discharge Consultation

Before you are officially discharged, you will normally be seen by your angioplasty physician or nurse for a pre-discharge consultation. Now is the time to ask more questions. You will obviously want to know how successful your angioplasty was, and what are the chances of your angina returning in the future. You will also want to know what to do in the event of an emergency. Once you have asked your questions, your physician or nurse will have lots of advice and information for you (some of this will be covered in Chapter 10). It is often a good idea to have a friend or relative present at this time simply as another pair of ears. Try writing things down, as well, to help you remember what you have been told.

Leaving the Hospital

Before you rush out of the hospital you might find the following checklist useful, to make sure that you have everything you need.

CHECKLIST – LEAVING THE HOSPITAL	✔
• Prescriptions	○
• Contact name & number in case of emergency	○
• General information package (groin care, etc.) including a list of dos & don'ts	○
• Someone to drive you home (you won't be allowed to drive for 24 hours after the surgery)	○
• Follow-up appointment (if applicable)	○
• Your personal items	○
• This book!	○

What Happens Next?

Once you are discharged you can go home, relax, and concentrate on making your recovery.

Chapter 10

recovering at home

What Happens in this Chapter

- Dealing with medication
- Care of your wound (at home)
- What to do in an emergency
- Guidelines for getting back to work
- Exercise, sex, driving, and flying
- Follow-up visits to your doctor or clinic

The first few days after your heart cath can feel like an uphill struggle. But be assured you will feel healthy again. By following a few simple guidelines and gradually increasing your activity, you will find that life soon starts to feel more normal.

Your First Day Back Home

Once you get out of the hospital, don't overdo things. Give your body time to adjust. Everyone is different so there are no absolute rules—except listen to your own body and do things within your own limits. Here is a useful list to remind you what you should, and should not, be doing.

[KEY POINT]

DO...

- Take it easy
- Get plenty of sleep
- Start a "heart healthy" diet
- Contact your physician immediately if you have an adverse reaction to your medication, such as a rash
- Plan an exercise routine
- Try some self-help techniques, such as relaxation or massage
- Try to keep stress to a minimum
- Quit smoking

DON'T...

- Rush back to work
- Do any heavy lifting or strenuous exercise
- Assume that since your angioplasty was successful, you can now return to your previous unhealthy diet and heart-unhealthy habits
- Forget that your groin will take 10 full days to heal
- Forget to take your medication
- Allow yourself to get stressed
- Continue to smoke

For advice on diet, exercise, and relaxation, see Chapter 11

Changes to Your Medication

Your medication may or may not be changed following your procedure. Some physicians may reduce your angina medication immediately after a successful angioplasty because your angina is greatly improved. More commonly, your medication is not changed until your first visit to your cardiologist, approximately 4 to 8 weeks after your angioplasty. He or she may then decide to reduce your medication based on a number of factors (see More Detail box).

Don't be surprised if you leave the hospital on more medications than you were on when you arrived. If you had a stent inserted into your blood vessel during your angioplasty, you will definitely be sent home on

> "I didn't let my heart problems stop me from doing what I wanted, but I'm cautious. If I feel any signs, I listen carefully to my body. All heart patients should learn to be in tune with their body."
>
> **Arni Cohn**

[MORE DETAIL]

Which Pills?

After your angioplasty, your physician will prescribe long-term medication based on the following factors:

- How you feel
- How quickly you return to normal
- Whether you need medication for other medical conditions, for example, high blood pressure
- Your cardiac risk factors
- Whether you had a stent inserted into your blood vessel

KEY POINT

Make sure you know exactly what medicines you should be taking and that you have a sufficient supply of tablets to take when you get home. You may find the diary pages at the back of this book useful for keeping a record of your medications.

clopidogrel (Plavix) for several months.

Your cardiologist may also decide that you are not taking enough medicine to stop your heart disease from getting worse. He or she may start you on medicine to reduce your blood cholesterol, lower your blood pressure, and help with heart failure, or, if you were on these medications before, the dose may be increased.

It is important that any physician who treats you knows about *all* the medications that you are on—not just drugs for your heart, but all medicines—including those that you buy over the counter without a prescription (for instance, herbal remedies, supplements, drugstore pain relievers). As the number of drugs you take increases, so do the chances of side effects from interactions between them. Remember that even complementary remedies such as herbal medicines have drug-like effects on your body and may interact with medicines that your doctor has prescribed for you, so be sure to tell him or her about them.

Caring for Your Incision

Your groin (or wrist) will be checked one last time before you leave the hospital. It is a good idea to take a shower rather than a bath on the first day after your angioplasty to reduce the risk of your groin or wrist starting to bleed again. It is also worthwhile checking your groin or wrist for signs of oozing or swelling every now and again, especially if you start to feel any pain in the area. Be prepared for a small amount of bruising. This is more common after angioplasty, due to the blood-thinning drugs that you received. It is sometimes difficult to decide between normal bruising and bruising that needs medical attention. In general, contact your doctor for any bruise associated with swelling or pain down the leg (rather than just simple discomfort), or a fever.

Physical Activity

It is normal to expect some discomfort from the site of your incision because your blood vessel will take 7 to 10 days to heal completely. If you had a heart cath or angioplasty via your groin, you should avoid strenuous exercise and heavy lifting for a week or two. If you have a physically demanding job, this may be a major inconvenience, but it pays to be careful at this stage because a return visit to the hospital as a result of bleeding would be even more inconvenient. If you had your heart cath or angioplasty via your wrist, you do not need to be as careful, but you may feel discomfort if you do activities that put strain on your wrist, such as tennis, golf, gardening or strenuous maneuvers, such as opening and closing windows.

Once your incision site has healed, regular exercise should be your top priority. Exercise is an essential part of your recovery and is one of the best therapies for your heart. It's a good idea to set goals for yourself and you might find it helpful to actually write them down (for instance, in the diary at the back of this book). Try to include exercise in your everyday routines. Walk up stairs instead of taking the elevator. Walk to the corner store or park (or gym) instead of using the car. Even when you are sitting down watching television, you can still do exercises such as leg lifts. Gradually, you will build up your stamina and, with a sensible exercise program, you should be able to achieve more and more—and feel better and better.

Pain or Breathlessness—What Do You Do?

If at any time you start to feel pain, short of breath, or your chest starts to feel "tight" STOP WHAT YOU ARE DOING IMMEDIATELY. It is NOT normal to experience breathlessness, central chest pain, or pain radiating down your left arm. If the pain does not go away, use your nitroglycerin under your tongue as directed by your physician. If after 3 doses you do not feel relief, call 911 to be taken to the nearest emergency room. This is just a precaution, in case your coronary artery has suddenly blocked since you left the hospital.

When you leave the hospital, your information package will include a telephone number for you to contact for help or advice regarding any other problems or questions you may have.

Sexual Activity

Once at home you can quickly resume a normal sex life, although it's a good idea to take it easy for the first week or two. It is not uncommon to feel very uneasy about resuming a normal sex life with your partner, especially if you have had a heart attack. In fact, sexual intercourse isn't as hard on your heart as you may think. It has been calculated that the effort required is roughly equivalent to walking up two flights of stairs. General advice is to resume lovemaking when both you and your partner feel ready. You may find the American Heart Association guidelines helpful (see More Detail box).

Affairs of the Heart —Sex After a Heart Attack

[MORE DETAIL]

The American Heart Association gives the following suggestions for lovemaking after a heart attack. These tips are also useful for people with angina.

- Choose a time when you are rested, relaxed, and free from stress brought on by the day's schedules and responsibilities.
- Wait 1 to 3 hours after a meal to allow it to digest.
- Select a familiar, quiet setting where you are unlikely to be interrupted.
- Take medicine before sexual activity, if prescribed by the doctor.
- Take it easy. Allow adequate time for foreplay, both to get your heart going gradually and to recapture some intimacy after spending time apart.

If you experience a rapid heartbeat or have difficulty breathing for 20 or 30 minutes after intercourse, have angina pain, or feel very tired the next day, consider slowing the pace down a bit.

In time, the partner who has had a heart attack or heart surgery is usually able to resume the same activity level as before (if not more so).

Driving

There is no law against driving immediately after a heart cath or an angioplasty, but most hospitals will recommend that you allow time for your groin to heal. The rule of thumb is that you can start to drive 2 to 3 days after your heart cath, although your physician may suggest a longer or shorter wait.

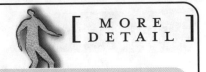

Flying

The recommendations on how soon after your angioplasty you can fly are determined more by medical insurance companies than physicians. Although you will probably be able to sit comfortably after a couple of weeks, you should check with your insurers about any rules they may have.

Returning to Work

> "It was several months before I felt really chipper again."
>
> **William Brumitt**

If you have a sedentary job, you can return to work very quickly after your heart cath or angioplasty. If your work involves either strenuous exercise or heavy lifting, you should wait approximately 10 full days before going back to work, to avoid triggering angina. If you have a *very* strenuous job (a firefighter, for example), it may be wise for you to be checked out by your family doctor or cardiologist before you return to work. He or she may wish to send you for an **exercise test** (see Glossary) to assess your cardiac condition before giving you the "all clear."

Follow-up Visits

Your primary care physician will have received a full report from the hospital and you will visit him or her 2 weeks after your procedure. You will also visit your own cardiologist 4 to 8 weeks after your angioplasty, or as directed. The reason for this is to allow him or her to check that you are generally well, to examine your groin (or wrist), and perhaps to confirm that it is safe for you to return to work, if you're still off. You may also need a repeat prescription for any new medications prescribed to you. The number of medicines you are taking may be reduced or increased according to your needs.

The number of times you need to visit a cardiologist or your primary care physician after these visits depends on how complicated your angioplasty and recovery are.

If you are feeling well, don't expect to be offered a further heart cath to "prove" that your heart cath worked. Most cardiologists are guided by their patients' symptoms: if you don't have any angina symptoms, you are unlikely to undergo any more testing, unless you are part of a clinical trial.

If your physician does recommend any tests, these will be similar to the ones you had before your heart cath. You *may* be asked to do an exercise test around 1 month after your angioplasty, with or without a **nuclear perfusion scan** (see Glossary). This tends to be done among patients with more complex heart disease so a re-blockage can be detected even before symptoms appear.

You may also need to have regular blood tests as a precaution, depending on your medications.

If your angina returns, contact your primary care physician or cardiologist so that you can be further evaluated. Diabetics are sometimes automatically re-tested every 2 years because they aren't always aware of their angina.

Beyond 9 Months

If you are well 9 months after your angioplasty, your return visits to your cardiologist or primary care physician should become less frequent. Unless you have other medical problems, you will only need to see your physician one or twice a year for routine follow-up. The emphasis now changes from looking after your symptoms to trying to prevent future problems.

What Happens Next?

> "I think that's the most important thing in terms of your recovery—to know what happened and what they're doing now and what you're going to anticipate. You recover faster if you understand what's going on and you can also avoid some mistakes along the way."
>
> **William Brumitt**

Once you have recovered from your angioplasty and things have returned to normal, you will, we hope, feel better than ever before. It's important to realize, though, that your heart disease has not been cured. Your angioplasty has only bought you time—time to take stock of your life, time to realize that your heart is in your hands. If you want to change your life, the next chapter shows you how.

Chapter 11

how you can help yourself

What Happens in this Chapter

- Lifestyle shifts that can transform your future
- Cardiac rehabilitation
- Changing your diet—the simple and easy way
- Exercising your way forward
- Supplements and herbal medicines
- Massage, visualization, acupuncture, relaxation
- The science of complementary therapies

It is a common misconception that angioplasty is a cure for heart disease and that it removes the disease from your coronary arteries. In fact, neither angioplasty nor heart bypass surgery stops your heart disease from gradually getting worse. A combination of factors contributed to your heart disease, and a combination of treatments is the only effective way forward. This includes a long-term commitment to exercise, dietary modification, and discontinuing tobacco products. Correcting only some of your risk factors, while ignoring others, will not work.

Healing Your (Whole) Self

IN THIS CHAPTER WE WILL LOOK AT WAYS IN WHICH YOU CAN improve your heart health through exercise and diet. We will also explore techniques such as visualization and relaxation, and other complementary therapies that you can use to help you prepare for your angioplasty procedure and take control of your life afterward.

Most of the therapies mentioned use a holistic approach to health. The word "holistic" comes from the Greek word *holos* meaning "whole." Holistic health care involves treating the whole person and not just one isolated body part or one risk factor. When you are considering what you can do to help yourself, think of healing your whole self and not just your heart.

[SELF-HELP]

Help Yourself to a Healthy Heart

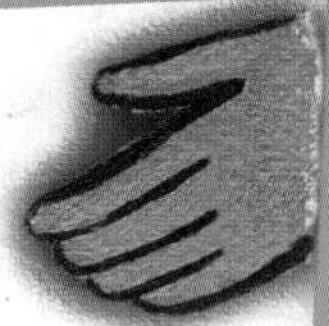

The "big four" (M.E.D.S.)

- **M**anage stress
- **E**xercise
- **D**iet
- **S**top Smoking

Some people also find these approaches helpful:

- Vitamins and supplements
- Herbal medicines (**used under medical supervision**)
- Visualization and relaxation techniques
- Massage, therapeutic touch, and acupuncture

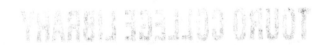

Cardiac Rehabilitation

Cardiac rehabilitation ("cardiac rehab") is a support program aimed at returning heart patients to an active, healthy life. Most programs begin around 1 to 3 months after your angioplasty and require a referral by your family doctor or cardiologist. The hospital will give you all the information you need about cardiac rehab before you go home. Joining a cardiac rehab program is one of the best things you can do for your heart—and yourself.

Cardiac rehabilitation involves several classes, spread out over a few months. The first, intensive part of the program involves a multidisciplinary team of physicians, exercise physiologists, nurses, occupational therapists, social workers, physical educators, lab technologists, and support staff. They will work out where you are now, and where you need to get to, and design an exercise and lifestyle program tailored to your own needs.

Studies have shown that patients who attend cardiac rehab have better recoveries than those who don't. The most important feature of cardiac rehab is the support that you will receive. Adjusting to your new life may be difficult, both physically and emotionally, and you may find that even family members can't always say or do just the right things. The team at cardiac rehab, and the other patients in the program, understand what you are going through and can give you exactly the right kind of advice and support for a healthy and happy recovery.

Healthy Lifestyle and Heart Disease

The old adage "you are what you eat" holds a great deal of truth, particularly when it comes to heart disease. Heart disease is a disease of overfed countries. It is important to take a step back, take a good look at your diet, and plan out what improvements you should make.

> "You have to drive the recovery and rehabilitation exercise. I went on a 9-month program designed to change your lifestyle and work you hard. The idea was a permanent change, to select a different road. I saw tremendous denial by other participants who thought they could cheat a bit."
>
> **Arni Cohn**

Many studies have shown that healthy eating can stop your heart disease from getting worse and, in combination with exercise and weight loss, may even reverse it. However, it must be a long-term commitment. Improving your diet for only a short period of time will make no difference to the health of your heart because atherosclerosis—the artery-hardening process that causes heart disease—is a chronic (long-term), not an acute (short-term), disease.

Changing the eating habits of a lifetime can be hard, especially if you aren't very confident in the kitchen, so get some help. Most hospitals can refer you to a dietician. Your cardiac rehabilitation program will also give you plenty of encouragement and practical advice.

What Is a "Heart Healthy" Diet?

Healthy eating involves eating a well-balanced diet containing foods from all the main food groups. No one food group alone can provide you with all the necessary nutrients needed to maintain health.

Fruit and Vegetables

There is plenty of evidence to show that a diet rich in fruit and vegetables helps to protect against, and potentially reverse, cardiovascular disease. Fresh fruit and vegetables are high in nutrients and fiber and low in calories. The exact reasons why they protect against heart disease is unknown. Part of the reason may be that a diet rich in high-fiber foods is likely to contain less saturated fat, a major cause of heart disease (and obesity, another risk factor for heart disease). It is also likely that there are active ingredients within fresh fruit and vegetables that help the body fight disease, including heart disease. The active ingredients are unknown, so beware of expensive supplements in health food shops that claim to be full of them. Try to eat at least five servings of fruit and vegetables each day and, if possible, eat organic produce and what is currently in season because these may be fresher and contain more nutrients.

Fiber

Most of us don't eat enough fiber, so it makes sense to boost this important part of your diet. This should help to reduce your cholesterol level and, because fiber fills you up without adding calories, it will also help to reduce your calorie intake and lower your body weight. You can get more fiber by incorporating plenty of fresh fruits and vegetables, as well as whole grains, nuts, and cereals (oatmeal, wheat germ, whole oats, etc.) into your diet.

Fats

When you're trying to choose heart-healthy food, it can get pretty confusing trying to sort out what you're meant to be doing about those fats. Dietitians now keep the advice simple: reduce your fat intake overall and *especially reduce saturated fats*. The easiest rule of thumb for managing this is to avoid products high in animal fats—all those hamburgers and hot dogs. The reason for this is that most animal fat is saturated fat.

"You have to work at it. Exercising, losing weight, changing diet, it's hard. A positive attitude is the best thing."

Robert (Bobby) Frew

If you wish to eat dairy produce, try to stick

with the lower-fat or non-fat products. These would include skim or 1-to 2-percent-fat milks, low-fat yogurt, and low-fat cheeses. Try using polyunsaturated or monounsaturated margarines for spreading on baked potatoes, bread, or other baked goods, and olive or canola oils for dressings, sauces, and frying.

How Low Do You Go?

There is a scientific debate raging, particularly in the U.S., over whether very low-fat diets (containing around 10 percent of calories from fat) can actually reverse heart disease. Some studies appear to support this idea, while others seem to show that once you get down to a certain point (about 25 percent), there is no further benefit gained from reducing fat. The debate will no doubt continue to get more interesting, but in the meantime, the advice is to aim for about 30 percent of calories from fats (many people find that hard enough), and reduce saturated fats and trans fats.

"Don't kill yourself if you don't follow-through 100 percent. Just try harder next time round."

Arni Cohn

Protein Sources

Use a variety of protein sources such as fish, soy products, lean meat, poultry, and legumes. If you do eat meat, stick to lean cuts and small portions. There is good evidence to show that eating at least one portion of oily fish per week (such as mackerel and sardines) has a heart-protective role in coronary heart disease (see Omega-3 fatty acids, page 113).

Beans, nuts, and legumes are great sources of protein and thus can be used as an alternative to fatty meats, as can soy products. Nuts and seeds also contain polyunsaturated fats (the "good" fats).

Salt

It is a good idea for all heart patients to limit their salt intake. Prepared foods, processed foods, and take-out type foods are generally high in salt. The current recommendation is about half a teaspoon of salt per day. Ask your doctor before using a salt substitute, which may contain too much potassium for your heart.

[KEY POINT]

Diets are hard, so let's keep the rules simple. Eat much more fiber, fruit, and vegetables and significantly reduce your total fat intake, especially saturated fats.

Alcohol

Recent studies have suggested that moderate alcohol intake (1 to 2 glasses of wine per day) may in fact reduce further heart attacks and may even be beneficial long-term for patients with heart disease. This advice should be weighed against the risk of overindulgence and also the alcohol's effect on the liver and other organs. Nevertheless, there is growing evidence that at least a small amount of wine drinking may be beneficial due to its antioxidant effects.

However, remember that alcohol is also high in calories and thus contributes to weight gain, so moderation is key. Avoid alcohol

What is a Drink?

[MORE DETAIL]

American guidelines on healthy alcohol consumption suggest that women should have no more than one drink, and men no more than two, per day.
1 drink =
4-oz glass of wine = 12-oz. bottle of beer = 1.5 oz of 80-proof spirits

completely while you are taking prescription pain medication or if you have raised triglyceride levels in your blood. Some heart medications should not be combined with alcohol: it is best to check with your pharmacist if you are unsure. If your doctor allows alcohol, limit your intake to 1.5 ounces of liquor, 1 beer, or 4 ounces of wine per day.

[SELF-HELP]

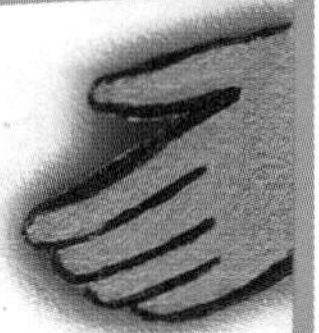

Help Yourself to a Healthy Diet

The following are some tips to help you eat your way to health:

- Take a heart-healthy cooking course. It will be fun, you'll meet other people in the same position as you, and you'll learn how food can be delicious as well as healthy.
- Load up on fruit, vegetables, and fiber at every meal. That way you'll have less room for fatty foods.
- Try to use fat-free broths instead of gravy.
- If you eat meat, each portion should be no bigger than the palm of your hand.
- Watch those "low-fat" bakery and dessert items. They are often very high in sugar, so you'll put on weight—which is also bad for your heart.
- Be aware of hidden saturated fats. Not all food labels list the saturated fat content. Be particularly suspicious of baked goods and pre-prepared meals.
- Avoid deep-fried foods. They are usually high in saturated fat or they may have a lot of **trans fats** (hydrogenated vegetable oils), the worst kind of fat for your heart.

Check Your Weight

It's hard, we know it is, but if you have heart disease, achieving and maintaining a healthy body weight is *essential*. Weight gain is associated with an increased risk of coronary artery disease and stroke. If you lose weight you may also reduce your blood pressure. The more gradual your weight loss, the greater the chance that the weight will stay off. "Crash diets" are an unsafe way to diet and, in the majority of cases, the weight will be regained. A consultation with a registered dietitian can help you work out what your ideal weight should be and help you set goals to achieve it. Keeping to the healthy diet guidelines above may be all that is needed to shed the extra pounds.

Check Your Blood Pressure

High blood pressure is the "silent killer" because it usually has no symptoms but makes your heart disease worse. If you have heart disease, you will almost certainly be taking blood-pressure-lowering medication, but you can further reduce your blood pressure with lifestyle modifications, in particular, losing some weight and reducing your salt intake.

Check Your Cholesterol

The most important thing you can do to lower your cholesterol, in addition to taking your cholesterol-lowering medicine, is to reduce the amount of saturated fat that you eat. There is also some evidence that soluble fiber, found in foods such as oatmeal, can lower blood-cholesterol levels.

Cigarette Smoking

There is overwhelming evidence that smoking is, without question, disastrous for the health of your heart. Chewing tobacco

[SELF-HELP]

Use the diary pages of this book to record and track your lifestyle goals. You can also use them to keep track of all your medications, including complementary medications.

[KEY POINT]

It's never too late to give up smoking.

"With exercise I kept my blood pressure normal for years. I learned to walk at a proper pace so as not to stress myself. I now walk a minimum of 6 hours a week. If I walk more I don't get credit for it, but if I walk less I have to make up for it next week."

T. Hofmann

products should also be avoided. The good news is that it is never too late to stop. Your risk of a heart attack or death falls rapidly once you stop smoking—by as much as 40 percent, according to one study. There is advice and support available to help you give it up. Some patients find the use of nicotine patches and gum helpful during the early phases of nicotine withdrawal. Talk to your primary care physician, cardiologist, or cardiac rehabilitation program.

Exercise

We all know about it, we've all done it (some of us still do it), not many of us do enough of it, and we all know how good it is for us.

Exercise is essential. There are no alternatives to it and you alone are responsible for doing it, since no one can do it for you.

Get a Helping Hand

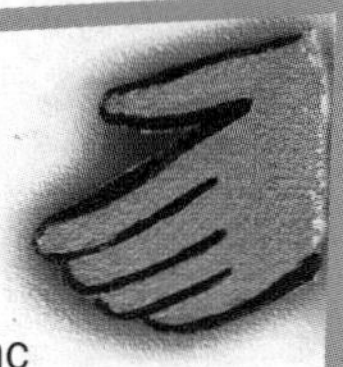

We strongly recommend that you enrol in a cardiac rehabilitation program, which will give you specific targets to aim for, general support, help, and advice based on your individual needs (see page 101).

Exercise can play a huge role in your recovery and long-term well-being. It can help you lose weight, it may lower your blood pressure, and may even stimulate new blood vessels to grow in your heart. Choose a sensible exercise program that suits you. You should aim for 30 minutes of moderate exercise at least 3 to 5 days of the week. Examples of moderate activities include cycling, fast walking, and swimming.

Stress Management

Our lives today contain enormous amounts of stress. Stress is the body's "fight or flight" response with nowhere to go, so the burden that stress places upon the body is huge. It acts as a silent and slow-acting body debilitator—almost like a disease in itself when it is left unattended. It can be years before we realize just how much stress we are under. It can take years, again, to actually recognize that we need to do

> "During the day I sit down for 2 or 3 minutes and internalize to see if I'm doing okay. If I've gone 2 or 3 hours without doing that, I know it mentally—I stop and relax and pull back, take a couple of deep breaths and say, 'How am I feeling?'"
>
> **Arni Cohn**

something about it. Even if we try to ignore stress, our bodies are extraordinarily clever at giving us warning signs that we are overdoing things. It is essential that you learn to recognize these signs and do something about them.

[KEY POINT]

Stress is potentially dangerous for heart health. However, there are many simple ways to deal with it. The key is to find a method of stress management that you feel comfortable with, to provide relief for your heart (and your head!).

Following are a few ideas that you might like to consider to control or manage your stress. See also Relaxation, Meditation, and Massage (pages 115–116).

Go for a Walk

You may not feel like it at the time, but once you get outside a walk can do wonders for clearing your head and lowering your blood pressure.

Deep Breathe

Sit down somewhere quiet (even if it means sitting in the washroom), and inhale and exhale slowly and deeply. As you breathe out, try to imagine all your anger or frustrations being blown out with your breath. Say to yourself, "I do not need this stress, my health is more important." Repeat this to yourself a few times before you go back to what you were doing.

Try to Avoid Arguments and Conflict

Avoiding a fight may be easier said than done, but nothing raises the blood pressure more effectively than a heated argument. Once again, ask yourself if the issue that is making you angry or frustrated is more important than your health. Is it possible to wait a few minutes or hours when all those involved in the conflict have calmed down? Perhaps then the issue at hand can be discussed more rationally and quietly.

Get Plenty of Sleep

Lack of sleep can only add to the stresses of the day. You can improve your chances of a good night's rest by

- not having caffeine after 4pm
- going to bed at the same time every night
- trying to sleep only when you're tired
- having a comfortable mattress
- buying some earplugs if your partner snores
- sleeping in a cool, dark, quiet room

Find a Hobby

Outdoor hobbies such as gardening are particularly helpful for stress. They can re-focus your mind and stop you from thinking about things that make you feel stressed.

Take Your Watch Off

Our lives are ruled by time. How many times in a day do you look at a clock or a watch? Find a day when you have nothing planned, take your watch off, and spend the day doing what you want, according to how you feel. Eat when you are hungry, rest when you feel tired, and fill in the rest of the time your way. You will be amazed at how re-energizing this can be.

Vitamins and Supplements

If you eat a well-balanced diet (see pages 102–105), it should provide you with all the essential nutrients and vitamins you need to achieve optimum health. You should consider vitamins and supplements only if you are not able to maintain a well-balanced diet.

If you have ever walked into a store selling vitamins and dietary supplements you will know that it can be overwhelming and confusing. If you are considering taking a supplement, discuss this with your primary care physician or cardiologist. Remember that some supplements can interact with prescribed medications.

[KEY POINT]

It is essential to inform all people involved in your care what supplements and medicines you are taking to avoid the risk of dangerous drug interactions. Physicians need to know about all non-prescription medicines and supplements; complementary therapists need to know about prescription drugs.

Multivitamins

Studies have shown that high doses of multivitamins can be unhealthy for heart disease patients. If you are considering multivitamins, consult a qualified professional.

Vitamins C and E (the antioxidant vitamins)

Despite many scientific studies, there is still no clear-cut evidence that vitamin C and E supplements make any difference one way or another to heart disease patients. It seems that vitamin E at a dose of 100 to 400 IU daily, combined with a diet high in fruits and vegetables and plenty of exercise, *may* be beneficial in heart disease patients. For vitamin C, there is still no overwhelming evidence that it is beneficial as a treatment for heart disease when taken as a supplement. In fact, the Los Angeles Atherosclerosis Study recently showed that high doses of vitamin C (850 to 5,000 mg/day) may make matters worse. This study found that artery disease progressed *faster* in patients taking these high doses of vitamin C, than it did in patients who did not take vitamin C supplements.

So why did some studies show a benefit and others did not? One possible explanation of why the vitamin supplements were ineffective in some of the studies is that the patients were sticking to a healthy diet and receiving adequate vitamin C and E anyway, so the supplements were unnecessary.

Folic Acid, B6, and B12

There has been a lot of interest in these supplements as a treatment for heart disease because deficiencies in these vitamins can cause high blood levels of an amino acid, linked to cardiovascular disease, called **homocysteine**. Recent studies have shown that B vitamins can reduce re-blockages after angioplasty. However, there is not, as yet, evidence to show that these supplements prevent or reverse atherosclerosis. A better choice might be simply to eat more fruit and fresh vegetables.

Co-enzyme Q10

Co-enzyme Q10 is a naturally occurring enzyme found within the body tissues, particularly in the heart, liver, and pancreas. To date, there have been no substantial studies on humans to prove its benefit for treating heart disease when given as a supplement (despite what the Internet may tell you).

Omega-3 Fatty Acids

Omega-3 fatty acids have been shown to have a protective role in coronary heart disease. To obtain your omega-3s without supplements, eat at least two fatty-fish meals per week or incorporate flax seeds, flaxseed oil, fish-oil tablets, hempseed oil, canola oil, and nuts into your diet. Get medical advice if you are taking fish-oil supplements with blood-thinning drugs.

Herbs

Herbs have been used as medicines since the beginning of humankind, and many of today's prescription medicines are based on natural substances found in herbs. Although there are numerous herbs advocated for use in heart disease, clinical studies have only been carried out on a few. Hawthorn has the most overwhelming evidence that it works.

Hawthorn

In large, well-designed clinical studies similar to those carried out on prescription drugs, hawthorn has been shown to increase blood flow to the coronary arteries, strengthen the heartbeat, and decrease blood pressure. It also has antioxidant properties and minimal side effects. Hawthorn is widely used throughout Europe as a medicine for the heart, often in combination with conventional drugs. However, hawthorn can affect the blood levels of other drugs, such as digitalis, glycosides, beta-blockers, and other blood-pressure-lowering drugs.

Garlic

There is good scientific evidence that garlic can protect your heart. One study, published in the *Journal of the Royal College of Physicians and Surgeons of London* in 1994, showed that eating 1/2 to 1 clove of garlic per day can reduce cholesterol levels by as much as 12 percent. Other reputable studies have shown that it has a blood-thinning effect, by reducing the stickiness of platelets (see Glossary), and can reduce the stiffness of the main blood vessel of the body, the aorta, in elderly people.

Ginko Biloba

Ginko is not as well-researched as hawthorn and garlic, but there are a few studies that show it increases blood flow and is an effective treatment for some circulatory diseases. A recent review of all studies, published in the *American Journal of Medicine* in 2000, concluded that ginko is particularly beneficial for treating artery disease in the blood vessels of the legs.

Other Herbs for Heart Disease

Other herbs used to treat cardiovascular disease for which there is scientific evidence include Terminalia arjuna, a traditional Ayurverdic herb used for heart conditions since the sixth century B.C., and tumeric. A recent study published in the *International Journal of Cardiolology* showed that Terminalia arjuna has benefits for patients with heart failure. Tumeric appears to have anti-platelet, cholesterol-lowering, and antioxidant properties.

The following herbs have been traditionally used to lower blood pressure, although there are no reputable scientific studies to either prove or disprove their effectiveness: olive leaves, cramp bark, yarrow, dandelion leaves, lime flowers, and mistletoe.

Safety Note

If you are considering the use of herbs to assist you with your health, it is essential that you discuss this with your cardiologist beforehand and enlist the help of an experienced herbalist or naturopathic doctor.

Other Complementary Therapies

Relaxation

It is widely recognized within the medical profession that people who learn to relax can control symptoms and, in some cases, even reduce blood pressure or pain. Relaxation can be achieved in a number of ways, including meditation, yoga, deep breathing, a nice hot bath, or simply imagining yourself lying on a hot, sunny beach. The trick is finding ways to relax in your current anxious state. Many cardiac rehabilitation programs now teach relaxation techniques as an integral part of recovery and there are numerous tapes and books on relaxation, so check out your local bookstore.

Meditation

Sit in a quiet place, focus on your breathing, and find a word or phrase that you can say over and over again to yourself. For example, you might try phrases that rid you of negative feeling towards other people and help you to accept personal differences. Letting go of such destructive feelings will give you more energy to focus on your own health and well-being. You might also consider a meditation program such as Tai Chi.

Visualization

This is a form of meditation that involves using mental imagery to bring about the changes you wish for. The idea—a visual version of "positive thinking," which may explain its apparent success in some people—is to believe that the more clearly you can see your desired future, the more chances there are of it becoming true. An example would be to imagine your blocked artery, unblocked. Although your angioplasty will accomplish this, positive thinking may, indeed, help your long-term health. There are numerous studies showing the power of the mind in medicine. Visualization can be practiced alone or in groups, and it usually requires the help of a therapist or tapes.

Acupuncture

Acupuncture has been in use for over 3,500 years in China and involves inserting fine needles into the skin and underlying tissues. Acupuncture practitioners consider acupuncture to work by stimulating the "vital force" or *qi* (pronounced chee)—the spiritual, mental, emotional, and physical aspects of a person. Although science has neither proven nor disproven that acupuncture works this way, what we do know is that it can relieve angina and angina-type symptoms in some people.

Massage

Massage is the art of using the hands to stimulate the skin and muscles to bring about a feeling of comfort and to promote healing. The Bible, the Qur'an, and the Ayur-Veda all mention the use of massage. There are many forms of massage, including Swedish, shiatsu, aromatherapy, reflexology, and neuromuscular. It can be a very positive experience and is the perfect way to reduce stress.

The Science of Complementary Therapies

[MORE DETAIL]

Complementary therapies for heart disease are, *generally speaking,* not as widely researched as conventional drugs or surgeries, and the studies that do exist are often not up to the standard of conventional drug trials. This means that we don't always know about side effects or how people with different diseases might be affected, so be cautious. A therapy isn't safe just because it's "natural" (the natural world contains some of our most powerful poisons). There are, however, a surprising number of good studies and the science of complementary therapies always makes for fascinating reading. See Resources at the back of this book.

Chelation Therapy—Does It Work?

Chelation therapy has been in use for approximately 40 years in North America for many different chronic illnesses. Heart disease patients generally receive chelation therapy intravenously (into a blood vessel). The theory is that chelation agents improve circulation by removing undesirable elements such as calcium and toxic metals from the blood, thus helping to reduce disease in the walls of blood vessels.

Intravenous chelation therapy in heart disease is extremely expensive and there are currently *no* reliable clinical trials proving that it works, although a large study is now underway in the U.S. to see if it has benefits. If you are considering chelation therapy you should think about it carefully, given the potential for adverse side effects, the expense, and the lack of any documented benefits so far.

What Happens Next?

If you have heart disease, no drug or surgery will work by itself. Likewise, no complementary therapy should be considered an "alternative" therapy, that is, a replacement for medical intervention. A combination approach—medical therapy, diet, exercise, other complementary approaches—is going to give you the best chance of slowing your heart disease and, possibly, even reversing it. Be sure to always tell your doctor about any complementary treatment that you decide to undertake. Likewise, be sure to tell any complementary practitioner about your angioplasty.

> "It's best to be realistic. I have accepted that some things I won't change, and I've tried to work on everything else."
>
> **Arni Cohn**

You are now well equipped to take full control of your heart's health. In the next chapter we look at the long-term results of angioplasty and how you can decide whether the procedure worked for you.

Chapter 12

has my angioplasty worked?

What Happens in this Chapter

- How you might feel right away
- What you might expect as you recover from the procedure
- The long-term picture

The success of your angioplasty procedure will usually be judged by how you feel, both immediately afterward and in the 9 months that follow. The majority of patients find that angioplasty relieves most or all of their angina symptoms and that they have no long-term problems.

Immediate Results

PATIENTS DO NOT LEAVE THE CARDIAC CATHETERIZATION laboratory until the angioplasty has finished and the physician has achieved the best possible result. You will, therefore, know fairly quickly how successful your angioplasty has been. If your physician is busy after your procedure and is not able to discuss the results with you right away, the cath lab nurses often will.

The Recovery Period

Once you have arrived back on the ward or recovery bay, your nurses will repeatedly ask how you are and encourage you to report any symptoms of chest pain immediately. If you have no chest discomfort, you can assume that your procedure is, thus far, a success.

Exactly how much better you feel when you are out of bed and walking around will depend on the severity of your angina symptoms before your angioplasty. If your angina was previously brought on by very little exercise, then you should notice an immediate improvement.

> "It was interesting because they took a photo from the video screen before and after so I could see the blockage, then see it being cleared. It's a positively uplifting thing to see that."
>
> **Bill Hogarth**

If your symptoms were moderate in severity beforehand, for example, needing a brisk walk to bring on the pain, you will probably not notice any difference until you leave the hospital. If your angina was mild before the procedure, that is, brought on only by vigorous exercise, then you may have to wait some time before knowing how well your angina has responded to the angioplasty. This is because you will not be able to exercise until your groin has fully healed.

Partial Revascularization

In some patients it is not technically possible, or it is too risky, to remove all the blockages in the coronary arteries. This result is known as **partial revascularization**, in contrast to **total revascularization** where all the narrowings are successfully treated.

If this is true in your case, you may be told that your angioplasty has been successful on the blood vessels that were treated, but that it was not possible to deal with all the narrowings. Disappointing, perhaps, but you should still gain some benefit. Although you may still have angina, you may find that you can tolerate more exercise before symptoms start.

"The main difference afterwards was how often the angina happened, and how bad it was. It used to be really bad, four or five attacks daily, but now I just get it occasionally or if I forget to put on the patch. I do get tired more easily, but that's normal for getting older."

Mrs. C.V.

In the rare cases where a physician attempts angioplasty, but is not successful (for whatever reason), obviously the symptoms of angina will remain unchanged.

The First 9 Months

Once you leave the hospital, your doctor will judge the success of your angioplasty mainly on *how you feel*. This may sound pretty untechnical, but studies have shown that using hospital tests to monitor the response to angioplasty is usually no more helpful than just asking the patient about his or her symptoms.

> "If you're out of surgery, you're not dead. Don't sit there being morose. Take a deep breath, look around, and say, 'You know what? I'm here now. I feel better, I have an opportunity. Let me get ahead with it.'"
>
> **Arni Cohn**

The first 9 months are crucial because this is the window during which re-narrowing (or **re-stenosis**) of your coronary arteries is most likely to happen. Studies show that currently up to one-third of patients have some re-stenosis, so re-narrowing of the arteries can almost be considered normal. However, the important consideration for each patient is whether this means that angina symptoms return. This so-called **clinical re-stenosis** happens in 15 to 30 percent of patients who have had a stent inserted, and 30 to 40 percent of patients after balloon angioplasty alone. Patients with drug-coated stents experience less re-stenosis. If you are unlucky and this does happen to you, your original symptoms of angina will return.

What Happens Next?

If you experience angina after the first 9 months, it is probably due to narrowing in one of your other coronary arteries as your heart disease progresses. This is why it is important to understand the reasons that you developed angina in the first place and do your best to make lifestyle changes to improve your heart's health.

> [KEY POINT]
>
> **If you do not correct** your "cardiac risk factors," such as smoking, obesity, lack of exercise, and a high-fat diet, your other blood vessels may become blocked in the future.

Chapter 13

medications

What Happens in this Chapter

- The major medications for angina
- How they work and the main side effects
- How to find the right medication mix for you

You are the most important member of your own care team, and never more so than when it comes to medications. You should always understand why you are taking each medicine, how to take it correctly, and any possible side effects, so that you can help your physician find the best combination for you. Medications for treating angina include drugs to prevent your angina symptoms, to treat them when they do arise, and to stop your heart disease from getting worse.

What Drugs Do You Need?

IF YOU HAVE ANGINA, YOU HAVE PROBABLY BEEN prescribed several kinds of medicines. They have three purposes:

- To prevent (or at least reduce) the number of angina attacks that you have (beta-blockers, calcium channel blockers, and nitrates).
- To treat angina attacks if and when they occur (nitrates).
- To prevent the disease in your blood vessels from becoming worse (anti-platelet agents, anticoagulants, ACE inhibitors, lipid-lowering drugs, and anti-hypertensives).

The precise types and doses of drugs that your doctor has prescribed for you to prevent or treat your angina depend on how severe your symptoms are, whether you suffer from any other illnesses, and how likely you are to experience the side effects of a particular drug.

[KEY POINT]

If you have had a heart attack or have been diagnosed with heart disease, it is likely that you will remain on some drugs for the rest of your life.

Drugs that prevent your heart disease from getting worse are needed because neither angioplasty nor bypass surgery actually stops the progress of the disease. Therefore, even if you undergo angioplasty or bypass surgery, you will need to take one or more of these "preventive" drugs afterward—possibly for many years in the future. The full list of medications your physician will prescribe depends on many factors, including whether you have had a heart attack, have high blood pressure, or have some other heart problem.

Drugs for Angina

All drugs are classified into groups based on what they do and how they work. There are hundreds of drugs that treat diseases of the heart and blood vessels (so-called **cardiovascular drugs**). Drugs that you are likely to be given can be divided into the following groups:

Nitrates

Nitrates, such as nitroglycerin, are used to both prevent and treat angina attacks. They have been in use for more than 75 years. Nitrates widen blood vessels, thereby increasing blood supply to the tissues (including the heart muscle) and reducing the amount of work the heart needs to do.

Beta-Blockers

These drugs reduce blood pressure, heart rate, and the strength of the heart's contraction. As a result, the heart needs less oxygen. Beta-blockers have been used for more than 20 years.

Calcium Channel Blockers

Also called **calcium antagonists** or **CCBs**, these drugs relax the muscles around blood vessels, thus widening arteries and increasing the blood flow and oxygen delivery to the heart muscle. They have been available since the 1980s.

Angiotensin-Converting Enzyme (ACE) Inhibitors

ACE inhibitors are a relatively new class of drugs, mainly used to treat high blood pressure and heart failure. However, they have also been shown to prevent angina from getting worse, to prevent heart attacks and severe angina, and to strengthen the heart muscle after a heart attack. They block the production of a substance that constricts blood vessels, thereby widening blood vessels and increasing the amount of oxygen that gets to the heart.

Anti-Platelet Agents

Once a blood vessel is narrowed by atherosclerosis, a blood clot can form on the blockage, causing severe angina or a heart attack. Anti-platelet agents reduce the tendency of blood platelets to form blood clots. There are a number of different ones (see Medications Table on page 128) with different uses, depending on how potent they are. ASA (Aspirin) is a useful anti-platelet agent that can be taken every day. Angioplasty greatly increases the risk of blood clots, so just before your angioplasty you will be given a stronger anti-platelet agent, such as clopidogrel (Plavix). During the procedure itself, when the risks are greatest, you may be given a highly potent anti-platelet therapy through your vein, such as abciximab (ReoPro), one of a group of drugs called **glycoprotein IIb/IIIa inhibitors**. (For more information on these drugs, see pages 50-52.)

Anticoagulants

Anticoagulants also prevent blood from clotting through a different mechanism from the anti-platelet agents. You can take anticoagulants as preventive medicine, for example, warfarin (Coumadin), or be given one (such as heparin or bivalirudin) during your angioplasty.

Lipid-Lowering Drugs

Lipid-lowering drugs such as **statins** and **fibrates** reduce the level of cholesterol and other fats in the blood. This helps to prevent your heart disease from getting worse by slowing down or stopping further narrowing of your coronary arteries. Clinical studies show that lipid-lowering drugs can reduce the risk of having a heart attack by one-third.

Other Blood-Pressure-Lowering Drugs

Beta-blockers, calcium channel blockers, and ACE inhibitors (see page 125) all reduce blood pressure in addition to their benefits for angina. Other types of blood-pressure-lowering drugs, or **anti-hypertensives**, that you may be prescribed include the **diuretics** ("water pills") and **angiotensin-II receptor antagonists (ARBs**, for short).

[SELF-HELP]

Help Yourself to the Right Medications

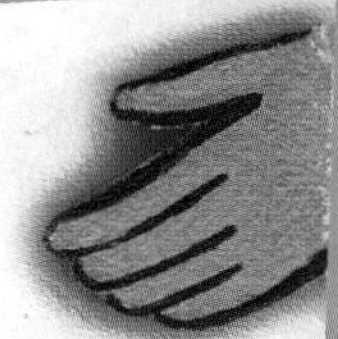

- Tell your doctor or nurse about any medication or food allergies.
- Always tell health professionals about other medications you are taking, such as complementary therapies, over-the-counter medicines, or supplements.
- Never stop a medication or cut the dose without first consulting your physician—even if you start to feel better.
- If you miss a dose, don't take double; just take the next dose as usual.
- Never take someone else's medication.
- Ask your doctor or pharmacist about possible side effects and report any unusual effects or reactions.
- Reorder medications before they run out to give your pharmacist time to reorder.
- Always carry a list of the medications that you are taking, and a note of what they are for. You may wish to use the diary pages at the back of the book.

Drugs Used in the Treatment of Angina

There are hundreds of cardiovascular drugs and only a selection is provided here.

Medications and Potential Side Effects

Drugs	Common side effects
Nitrates e.g., isosorbide-5-mononitrate (Imdur, ISMO, Monoket), isosorbide dinitrate (Dilatrate, Isordil, Sorbitrate), nitroglycerin (Minitran, Nitro-Bid, Nitro-Dur, Nitrolingual, Nitrostat, Transderm-Nitro, Tridil)	dizziness, fainting, headache, low blood pressure, irregular heart rhythms, nausea, blurred vision, sweating
Beta-blockers e.g., acebutolol (Monitan, Sectral), atenolol (Tenormin), labetalol (Normodyne, Trandate), metoprolol (Lopressor), nadolol (Corgard), pindolol (Visken), propranolol (Inderal)	contraction of the throat muscles, fatigue, dizziness, low blood pressure, sleep disturbances, slow heart rate, cold hands and feet, diarrhea, constipation, nausea or vomiting, impotence, skin discoloration, fever
Calcium channel blockers e.g., amlodipine (Norvasc), diltiazem (Cardizem, Cartia, Dilacor, Tiazac), felodipine (Plendil), nicardipine (Cardene), nifedipine (Adalat, Procardia), verapamil (Calan, Covera, Isoptin, Verelan)	headache, fast or slow heart rate, stomach upset, constipation, swollen tissues, dizziness, frequent need to urinate, palpitations, low blood pressure, flushing, tiredness, insomnia, muscle stiffness
ACE inhibitors e.g., benazepril (Lotensin), captopril (Capoten), enalapril (Vasotec), fosinopril (Monopril), lisinopril (Prinivil, Zestril), quinapril (Accupril), ramipril (Altace)	cough, low blood pressure, headache, dizziness, fatigue, nausea or vomiting, kidney problems, rash, altered sense of taste, swollen ankles, fever, joint pain
Anti-platelet agents e.g., abciximab (ReoPro), ASA (acetylsalicylic acid) (Aspirin), clopidogrel (Plavix), eptifibatide (Integrilin), tirofiban (Aggrastat)	dizziness, chest or stomach pain, headache, rash, diarrhea, vomiting, flushing, swollen ankles, joint pain
Anticoagulants e.g., bivalirudin (Angiomax), heparin (Hep-Lock), warfarin (Coumadin)	stomach pain, hair loss, blurred vision, rash, hives, itching, loss of appetite, diarrhea, skin discoloration, bruising
Statins e.g., atorvastatin (Lipitor), fluvastatin (Lescol), lovastatin (Mevacor), pravastatin (Pravachol), simvastatin (Zocor)	stomach problems, muscle pain and weakness, liver problems, visual disturbances, hair loss
Fibrates e.g., clofibrate (Abitrate), fenofibrate (Tricor), gemfibrozil (Lopid)	stomach problems, rash, weight loss, hair loss, headaches, nausea

The trade names of these drugs are based on information available at the time of publication. They may change. If in doubt, look for the generic name on your box of medication.

What About Side Effects?

All drugs have the potential to cause side effects. The goal is to avoid side effects or keep them to a minimum so that you don't notice them too much and they don't do any harm. Read the information that comes with your drugs or ask your pharmacist or physician about the possible side effects of your medication. See also the Table on page 128.

What Happens Next?

When you leave your doctor's office with a prescription, the next steps are up to you. Surprising as it may seem, many people with life-threatening conditions do not fill their prescriptions and, when they do, often fail to take the medication properly—or at all. Your medicines are part of your recovery process, so be sure to take them exactly as prescribed. Don't forget, too, that if you make lifestyle changes to improve your health, your doctor may be able to reduce the number or dose of medications that you take (see Chapter 11 for some help with this).

Chapter 14

the future of angioplasty

What Happens in this Chapter

- Taking part in a clinical trial
- Up-coming tools and techniques that could further improve the results of angioplasty

Patients already benefit from the technological strides that angioplasty has made in the last two decades. However, the procedure still has its limitations, so the quest for new and better techniques continues. Upcoming technologies that may soon become realities for patients include stents that patch tears in arteries and are self-absorbing, devices that prevent further blockage by freezing artery walls, and tools that sense when a blockage is about to rupture.

Clinical Trials and You

WHEN YOU ARE ADMITTED TO THE HOSPITAL FOR YOUR PROCEDURE, you may be asked to take part in a research trial for a new angioplasty technology or a new drug for use during angioplasty procedures.

If you are approached, carefully read the documents the research nurse (see page 139) will give to you before agreeing to anything. If you agree to take part, you will need to sign a written consent form. If you have any questions or want any more details before you sign, ask your physician or the research nurse before your procedure. If you still have lingering doubts about being involved, don't be afraid to say no. It will not count against you; your physician will continue to provide you with the care that is right for you.

Less is More: Trends in Angioplasty

The advances that have been made in angioplasty over recent years are part of a general trend for surgical procedures to be performed through smaller and smaller incisions. This increase in **key-hole** or **minimally invasive surgery** has been driven by patients and hospital administrators, as well as by physicians. Patients generally prefer minimally invasive surgery because the scalpel incisions leave smaller scars and allow for a quicker recovery and shorter hospital stay.

Angioplasty—being a minimally invasive technique—has always had the advantage over bypass surgery in that it involves less patient trauma, a faster discharge from the hospital, and a quicker recovery. Because of these advantages, angioplasty technology is here to stay and will continue to develop. The goal of angioplasty research is, first, to enable physicians to get better results by gradually overcoming some of the limitations of angioplasty (see page 43). The second goal is to help patients who are not currently suitable for angioplasty, such as patients with blockages that have been present for many years.

Recent Improvements in Angioplasty

The routine use of stents during angioplasty has improved both the short- and long-term results of the procedure. Emergency bypass surgery following angioplasty, which is usually needed if the blood vessel becomes blocked after the angioplasty balloon is inflated, has now fallen from as much as 3 percent to less than 1 percent of all procedures. The long-term picture has also improved: studies show that the risk of re-stenosis (with a return of your angina) after stent insertion is only 15 to 30 percent, as opposed to 30 to 40 percent with balloon angioplasty alone. The rate for re-stenosis with drug-eluting stents (see page 66) is so far even lower at only 4 to 8 percent.

Furthermore, improvements in both the design and construction materials of angioplasty equipment have significantly improved the performance of catheters, guide wires, balloons, and stents—and made them easier for physicians to use.

Finally, new blood-thinning drugs (see page 51) have reduced the frequency of blood-clotting problems and the occurrence of small heart attacks during angioplasty, without increasing the risk of major bleeding complications.

Covered Stents

Stents lined with a membrane made of Teflon were originally designed for angioplasty of heart bypass grafts. The plaques in this type of bypass graft crumble much more easily than in the heart's natural arteries, so there is a greater risk that portions of the plaque may fall away during the angioplasty procedure, block a blood vessel downstream, and cause a heart attack. Membrane-covered stents hold the plaque in place as the stent expands, preventing debris from escaping (see Figure 14–1).

Covered stents are also increasingly being used for angioplasty of the heart's own arteries, although they are not suitable for all blood vessels. These stents can help strengthen blood vessels with weak walls (**aneurysms**) and are useful for the emergency treatment of blood vessels that tear during the procedure.

Figure 14–1. A Covered Stent

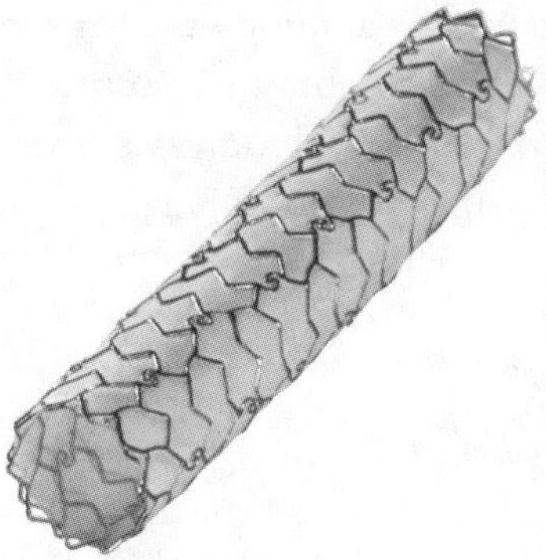

This special stent is, in fact, two stents with Teflon material sandwiched in-between. It is designed to reduce the risk of stray pieces of plaque blocking blood vessels downstream.

Self-Absorbing Stents

Self-absorbing stents slowly dissolve into a blood vessel after their insertion. These devices may improve the long-term results of stenting. They may also allow future bypass surgeries to be performed more easily because there is no metal meshwork to get in the way of the new bypass grafts. It is an interesting idea and a potentially exciting development for the future. However, there is only one self-absorbing stent currently under investigation and its long-term results are not yet known.

Thermography Catheters

Thermography catheters produce a thermal image—or temperature map—of blood vessels. Information from special temperature-sensing wires provides a real-time image that shows which parts of a blood vessel are too hot. If the temperature of a blood vessel is too high, cardiologists know that a blockage may be about to rupture and cause a heart attack. These high-risk areas in the blood vessel can then be treated with angioplasty and possibly a stent. Thermography devices are not yet approved for use in the United States.

Oxidation Catheters

Some treatments are being developed that aim to improve the results of angioplasty by temporarily boosting oxidation (the amount of oxygen) in the blood. During the angioplasty procedure, an oxygen-saturated fluid is flushed through the blood vessel, which makes its way to the heart muscle and helps reduce oxygen starvation (**ischemia**).

Cryogenic Catheters

There is a catheter under investigation that is designed to prevent re-stenosis by freezing the blockage (see Figure 14–2). A special balloon is expanded inside the blocked blood vessel, which is then cooled to below freezing. The temperature drop weakens the fatty blockage and allows it to be compressed evenly. It is hoped that this approach also permanently changes the elasticity of the artery's tissues, so that they won't recoil or re-stenose once they've been stretched.

Figure 14–2. PolarCath™ CryoPlasty™ System

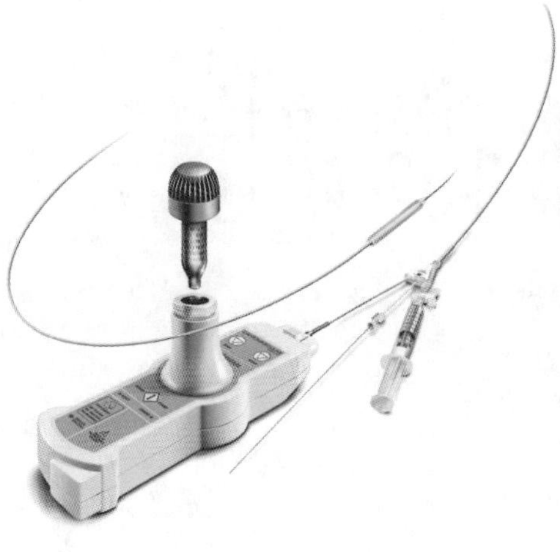

This experimental device uses a tiny balloon filled with super-cooled nitrous oxide, designed to open the blockage in the artery more easily and reduce the risk of renarrowing.

Chapter 15

who's who of hospital staff

What Happens in this Chapter

- Hospital staff you will meet
- A brief overview of their roles

When YOU GO IN THE HOSPITAL, YOU WILL ENCOUNTER A LARGE number of staff. Generally speaking, the hospital staff will be friendly and approachable. If you are dealing with them directly, they should introduce themselves and explain their role in your care. All employees wear an ID badge and you should feel free to ask staff members to identify their role in the hospital.

To add to the confusion, many of the hospital staff, from porters to doctors, wear white coats or "scrubs" (loose pants and tops), making it hard to figure out who's who. In addition, within the title of "doctor" or "nurse" are a number of different roles. For example, you may see a **fellow**, an **intern**, or an **attending cardiologist**. All are doctors, but all have varying levels of knowledge and ability. Or, you may see a **ward nurse**, an **angioplasty nurse**, a **nurse practitioner**, and a **research nurse**. Again, all are qualified nurses, each with a different role.

This chapter explains who is who in the hospital and what each person does.

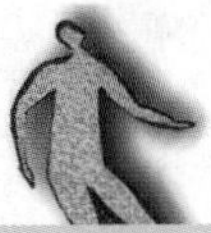

[MORE DETAIL]

Medical Staff	Mid-level Practitioners	Nursing Staff	Ancillary/ Support Staff
Attending cardiologist	Nurse practitioner	Cardiology staff nurse	Blood technician
Fellow	Physician assistant	Cath lab nurse	Cath lab technician
Intern		Research nurse	ECG technician
Medical student			Nursing assistant
Resident			Ward clerk/ receptionist

[KEY POINT]

Everybody you will meet in the hospital has a defined role. If you are not sure who somebody is, don't be afraid to ask.

Attending Cardiologist

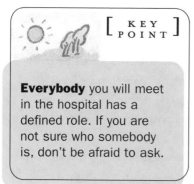

An experienced physician who has undergone considerable training in cardiology and who is now in a position to make independent decisions regarding patient care and treatment. The attending cardiologist is responsible for your overall care and for the decisions made by more junior staff.

Blood Technician

A person who is trained specifically to draw blood samples, usually from the arm.

Cardiology Fellow

Qualified internal medicine physician who is training in a speciality area such as cardiology.

Cardiology Staff Nurse

A qualified nurse who works in the cardiology patient care unit providing patient care. These nurses have a range of roles, depending on seniority and experience. They are responsible for your well-being and safety during your stay on the ward.

Cath Lab Nurse

A qualified nurse involved in everything from patient check-in to the completion of the procedure. He or she usually has several years of experience, primarily in the field of cardiology. The cath lab nurse may either assist the physician performing your angioplasty or help elsewhere within the cath lab. Alternatively, he or she may work at the monitoring station or in the recovery area. He or she may also play a part in patient education, discharge planning, and advice. If you have a question regarding the dates and times of your angioplasty, the cath lab nurse would be the person to contact.

Cath Lab Technician

A person who has a radiology background and sometimes works interchangeably with the cath lab nurses in their role within the cath lab.

ECG Technician

A person who is specifically trained to perform ECGs on the patient. He or she may also assist in other areas that require heart monitoring, such as assisting with exercise tolerance testing or Holter tape monitoring.

Medical Student

A person who is training to become a physician.

Nurse Practitioner

A registered nurse with advanced training who has completed a master's degree. He or she operates at a high level of competency and independence, performing physical examinations, providing patient education, and giving clinical support to the physicians.

Nursing Assistant

A person who has undergone training to assist nurses in patient care.

Physician Assistant

An advanced health care professional with a master's degree who functions at a high level of competency. He or she often performs physical exams, and provides technical and clinical support to the attending physician.

Research Nurse

A qualified nurse who specializes in research and whose role is to approach patients regarding possible participation in research studies. It is his or her job to supply the patient with information about the study, such as the commitment involved, the follow-up schedule, side effects, and potential complications. In some instances the research nurse is also responsible for collecting blood for the study (if it is needed) and seeing patients at follow-up appointments.

Resident or Intern

A junior doctor in training. He or she can specialize in a particular area, such as cardiology.

Ward Clerk or Receptionist

Usually the first person you will meet upon your arrival to the ward. He or she is responsible for organizing the administration of the ward. Often his or her role extends beyond this, depending on experience level.

Disclaimer: The above descriptions are intended as a general guide only. The roles of each type of staff member mentioned may differ slightly from hospital to hospital.

glossary

ACE inhibitor A drug used to treat hypertension and congestive heart failure, as well as to prevent heart attacks and worsening of angina.

Activated clotting time (ACT) A test of how much the blood has been "thinned" and how likely it is to clot.

Acute marginal branch One of the branches of the right coronary artery.

Acute myocardial infarction A heart attack.

Allen's test A test performed on the blood vessels in the wrist to check if the angioplasty can be safely performed via the radial artery in the wrist. This involves blocking the radial artery in your wrist and checking that your fingers are still receiving blood via the ulnar artery.

Anesthetic A drug used to numb an area of skin ("local") or put someone to sleep ("general").

Aneurysm An abnormal dilatation or widening of a blood vessel due to a weakness in its wall. It can occur in a coronary artery or in a groin artery after coronary angiography or angioplasty.

Angina Chest pain caused by lack of oxygen to the heart muscle.

Angiogram *See* Angiography.

Angiography A procedure involving the injection of X-ray dye into a blood vessel to produce an image of that vessel. An angiogram is the still or video image produced by angiography.

Angioplasty An operation that widens narrowed blood vessels.

Anti-anginal drugs Medication used to relieve or prevent symptoms of angina.

Anticoagulant A medication that "thins" the blood by blocking the activity of proteins involved in blood clotting.

Anti-platelet drug A medication that "thins" the blood by blocking the activity of small cell fragments in the blood called platelets.

Aorta The main blood vessel of the body, which carries oxygenated blood from the heart to the rest of the body.

Aortic stenosis Narrowing of the aortic valve, resulting in increased strain on the heart muscle as it tries to pump blood through the narrowed valve. This is a cause of angina and can be corrected by valve surgery.

Aortic valve The valve through which oxygen-rich blood leaves the heart before passing into the aorta.

Artery A blood vessel that carries oxygen-rich blood from the heart to the body tissues.

Atherosclerosis A disease that commonly narrows or blocks arteries anywhere in the body. It involves the development of a fatty, calcium-rich deposit on the inner wall of the arteries called plaque that gradually builds up over many years.

Balloon angioplasty An operation that widens narrowed blood vessels by inflating a tiny balloon inside the narrowed part of the vessel.

Beta-blocker A drug used to reduce blood pressure and/or prevent angina symptoms.

Brachial artery The artery in the elbow.

Bypass surgery *See* Coronary artery bypass graft.

CABG *See* Coronary artery bypass graft.

Calcification The hardening of tissues due to the accumulation of calcium within them.

Calcium channel blocker A drug used to reduce blood pressure and/or prevent angina symptoms.

Cardiac catheterization ("heart cath") A procedure in which a long tube or catheter is inserted into the heart via an artery in the arm or groin. Cardiac catheterization allows physicians to carry out procedures on the heart, such as coronary angioplasty, without opening up the chest wall.

Cardiac catheterization laboratory The X-ray room where coronary angiograms and angioplasties are performed in hospitals. Also known as the **cath lab**.

Cath lab *See* Cardiac catheterization laboratory.

Catheter A narrow tube that is inserted into a part of the body.

Cholesterol A type of fat that accumulates in the walls of diseased blood vessels.

Circumflex artery ("circ") One of the three main blood vessels of the heart. It supplies oxygen to the muscle on the left side of the heart.

Clinical trial A test (of a drug or procedure) that involves patients.

Closure device A piece of equipment used to repair (close) the small hole in the artery of the leg through which an angiogram or angioplasty was performed.

Conduits The tubes used to bypass narrowed or blocked arteries during coronary bypass operations. *See also* Grafts.

Coronary angiogram An angiogram performed on the coronary arteries.

Coronary angioplasty Angioplasty performed on the coronary arteries.

Coronary arteries The arteries that supply blood to the muscle of the heart itself. There are three main coronary arteries: the right coronary artery and the two branches of the left coronary artery.

Coronary artery bypass graft (CABG) The correct medical term for "heart bypass surgery" or "bypass surgery." This surgery is carried out to relieve angina by creating a bypass around blocked or narrowed coronary arteries. The bypass itself is a short length of artery or vein taken from the leg or chest and grafted onto the heart above and below the blocked artery.

Coronary artery disease Any disease involving the coronary arteries. Most commonly used to describe blockage of the coronary arteries due to atherosclerosis.

Cross-matching A laboratory test used to find out which type of donated blood is suitable to give a specific person for a transfusion.

Diagnostic test / procedure A test or procedure used to determine the cause of a medical disorder.

Diagonal artery One of the branches of the left anterior descending artery.

Directional atherectomy A method of removing diseased material from narrowed blood vessels by using a cutting blade mounted on the end of a catheter.

Dissection A tear in the blood vessel wall. This can be a complication after balloon angioplasty.

Doppler flow wire A special guide wire used during angioplasty to measure the blood flow in the vessel.

Drug-coated stents *See* Drug-eluting stents.

Drug-eluting stents Stents coated with medicine that prevents the artery from re-narrowing.

Echocardiogram (echo) An ultrasound image of the inside of the heart. Used to examine the size and function of heart structures, such as valves, and diagnose heart disorders. Usually performed by placing a transducer (probe) on the skin above the heart and is painless.

ECG *See* Electrocardiogram.

Electrocardiogram (ECG) A recording of the electrical activity of the heart. This can be useful for diagnosing angina or a heart attack.

Embolization Sudden blockage of a blood vessel due to passage of a foreign body through the bloodstream. In balloon angioplasty, it occurs when debris is released from diseased blood vessels.

Embolus A blood clot or piece of loose plaque that blocks a blood vessel.

Endothelium The normal lining of the inside of a blood vessel.

Exercise test A test for angina during which a patient walks on a treadmill with ECG wires attached to the chest, arms, and legs.

General anesthetic A drug or combination of drugs used to put a patient to sleep.

Glycoprotein IIb/IIIa inhibitors Special blood-thinning anti-platelet drugs used during angioplasty.

Graft The tube used in bypass surgery to re-route blood around blood vessel narrowings or blockages. It is usually taken from a blood vessel in the leg or chest.

Guide wire An essential piece of equipment used during every angioplasty operation. This is the first piece of equipment that is inserted along the blood vessel and across the blockage. Angioplasty equipment, such as balloons and stents, runs along the guide wire into the blood vessel.

Heart attack The sudden blockage of one of the heart's blood vessels, resulting in the death of a portion of the heart muscle.

Heart bypass surgery *See* Coronary artery bypass graft.

Heart cath *See* Cardiac catheterization.

Heart failure ("congestive" or "cardiac") The condition that results when the heart fails to pump blood properly through the system.

Hematoma A swelling resulting from a collection of blood under the skin usually caused by a broken blood vessel.

Hypertension High blood pressure.

Intensive care unit (ICU) A specialized ward that looks after severely ill patients or those who have had major operations.

Intravascular ultrasound (IVUS) A technique that involves taking pictures of the inside of a blood vessel with probes mounted on miniaturized catheters. IVUS provides more detail than angiography.

Invasive test A test in which part of a surgical tool enters the body.

Ischemia Lack of oxygen to the tissues. If ischemia lasts too long it can damage the tissue or even cause the tissue to die.

IVUS *See* Intravascular ultrasound.

Left anterior descending artery (LAD) One of the three main blood vessels of the heart. It supplies oxygen to the muscle at the front of the heart.

Left main coronary artery The most important blood vessel in the heart. It divides into the left anterior descending artery and the circumflex artery.

Left main disease Disease in the left main coronary artery. In severe cases bypass surgery is usually recommended, although angioplasty may sometimes be more appropriate.

Left ventricle The main pumping chamber of the heart.

Lipid-lowering therapy Medication to lower the levels of cholesterol and other fats in the blood.

Local anesthetic A drug that numbs the sensation of pain at the site of the injection.

Lumen The hollow space inside a blood vessel through which the blood flows.

Multiple-vessel disease Heart disease involving two or more main coronary arteries that supply the heart muscle.

Myocardial infarction A heart attack.

Nitrate A drug used to relieve or prevent angina symptoms.

Nitroglycerin The most commonly used nitrate drug.

Non-invasive test A test not requiring any equipment to be inserted into the body.

Nuclear perfusion scan A test in which a radioactive isotope is injected into the body to measure the flow of blood. This test is used to diagnose angina. It can be done in addition to, or before, an angiogram. This test is often used for people who are unable to exercise on a treadmill.

Obtuse marginal (OM) branch One of the branches of the circumflex artery.

Occlusion A blockage of a vessel.

Pacemaker The control center in the heart that determines how fast the heart beats. An artificial or temporary pacemaker is a wire that is inserted into the heart to control the heart rate.

Painless or "silent" ischemia Angina without symptoms of chest pain.

Partial thromboplastin time (PTT) A test to measure the clotting time of blood. If the blood is too thin, or not clotting enough, a patient is at risk for bleeding; if the blood is clotting too much, a patient is at risk for stroke or heart attack.

PCI *See* Percutaneous coronary intervention.

Percutaneous coronary intervention (PCI) The correct medical name for a treatment that takes place via a heart cath, such as angioplasty.

Pericardium The thin membrane that covers the heart.

Peripheral transluminal angioplasty (PTA) A procedure that widens blocked arteries in parts of the body other than the heart.

Peripheral vascular disease (PVD) Disease that blocks the blood flow in blood vessels not in the heart (e.g., the leg arteries).

Plaque The blockage responsible for narrowing blood vessels in atherosclerosis. A plaque is usually composed of tissue cells, fatty material, and, sometimes, calcium deposits. A complicated plaque is one that has become ulcerated (broken open), contains a blood clot, or is irregular in appearance. An uncomplicated plaque is usually a smooth narrowing in a blood vessel.

Platelets Small cell fragments in the blood that are essential for blood clotting.

Positive remodeling The response of a blood vessel to the development of atherosclerosis in its wall. In the early stage of disease, the blood vessel expands in an attempt to keep the lumen of the blood vessel open and the blood flowing normally through it.

Posterior interventricular or descending branch (PIV or PDA) One of the branches of the right coronary artery. It supplies blood to the inferior surface (bottom) of the heart.

Pressure wire A special guide wire used during angioplasty to measure the blood flow in the vessel.

Prognosis A prediction of the probable outcome of a disease and how likely recovery is.

Pseudo (false) aneurysm Not a true aneurysm (widening of a blood vessel wall), but a similar-looking swelling caused by a persistent leak in the wall. This is an occasional complication of coronary angiography or angioplasty at the point where the sheath was inserted into the groin or wrist.

PTA *See* Peripheral transluminal angioplasty.

PTT *See* Partial thromboplastin time.

Radial artery One of the two arteries in the wrist through which a heart cath and angioplasty can be performed.

Radio-opaque Visible on X-rays. Radio-opaque dye is used during coronary angiography and angioplasty.

Renal failure When your kidneys do not work properly.

Re-stenosis Re-narrowing of a blood vessel that was once widened.

Revascularization The restoration of blood flow into the heart muscle by either angioplasty or bypass surgery.

Right coronary artery (RCA) One of the three main blood vessels of the heart. It supplies oxygen to the muscle on the right side and underside of the heart.

Rotational atherectomy The removal of hard material such as calcium from narrowed or diseased blood vessels using a drill-like device. This is usually done at the same time as balloon angioplasty and stenting.

Sedative A drug that lowers the level of consciousness and makes the person feel tired or sleepy.

Sheath The short tube inserted into the blood vessel in the groin or wrist, through which longer tubes (catheters) are inserted and passed to the heart during coronary angiography or angioplasty.

Single-vessel disease Heart disease involving just one of the three main blood vessels supplying the heart muscle.

Stable angina Angina that is consistently brought on by exercise or stress and does not occur during rest or sleep.

Stenosis (plural: stenoses) A narrowing of an artery.

Stent A metal coil or tube used to keep a blood vessel fully open.

Stress test *See* exercise test.

Stroke Damage to the brain caused by either bleeding from a burst blood vessel in the brain or blockage by a blood clot.

Suture A stitch.

Temporary pacemaker wire A metal wire that is inserted into the heart via the leg, arm, or shoulder, to temporarily take over the heart's own pacemaker. It can be used during angioplasty if the heart rate slows down, causing a drop in blood pressure.

Thrombectomy A procedure carried out to remove a blood clot.

Thrombosis The process of blood clotting.

Thrombus (plural: thrombi) A blood clot that may block a blood vessel.

Transient ischaemic attack (TIA) A "mini-stroke" from which the person makes a full recovery.

Trans-radial approach Angioplasty performed via the wrist.

Treadmill test *See* Exercise test.

Triple-vessel disease Heart disease involving all three of the main blood vessels supplying the heart muscle.

Troponin A heart muscle protein that can be measured in a blood sample after a heart attack or episode of severe angina.

Ultrasound An imaging technique that uses sound waves.

Unstable angina Angina that develops for the first time, suddenly becomes more severe, or occurs at rest.

Vein A blood vessel that carries oxygen-poor and carbon dioxide-rich blood back to the heart and lungs.

resources

Heart Health Information

So You're Having Heart Bypass Surgery
By Tracey Colella RN, Suzette Turner RN, Bernard Goldman MD, and Brett Sheridan MD. John Wiley & Sons Inc, 2003. ISBN 0-470-83346-7

American College of Cardiology
Heart House
9111 Old Georgetown Road
Bethesda, MD 20814–1699
Tel: (800) 253–4636, ext. 694 or (301) 897–5400
Fax: (301) 897–9745
Clinical statements and guidelines, educational material, media, journals, and news on cardiology.
http://www.acc.org

International Task Force for Prevention of Coronary Heart Disease
Assessing and preventing heart disease.
http://www.chd-taskforce.de

The Mended Hearts, Inc.
7272 Greenville Avenue
Dallas, TX 75231
Tel: (214) 706–1442
1–888–HEART99 (1–888–432–7899) (US only)
Support for heart disease patients.
http://www.mendedhearts.org

National Heart, Lung, and Blood Institute (NHLBI)
Information about heart and blood vessel disorders, including angina and heart attacks.
http://www.nhlbi.nih.gov/health/public/heart/index.htm

Yale Heart Book
Detailed articles about heart disease and its prevention and treatment.
http://www.med.yale.edu/library/heartbk

Stress and Relaxation Information

Directory of Stress Management Resources
Tests, tips, and resources on stress management.
http://www.stresstips.com/directory

VirtualPsych
Includes a large section on stress management.
http://www3.telus.net/virtualpsych

Nutrition and Fitness Information

Food & Nutrition Information Center
Agricultural Research Service, USDA

National Agricultural Library, Room 105
10301 Baltimore Avenue
Beltsville, MD 20705–2351
Tel: (301) 504–5719
Government-sponsored organization that provides information on dietary supplements, food composition, dietary guidelines, and many more nutrition topics.
http://www.nal.usda.gov/fnic/

Guidelines for Personal Exercise Programs
Developed by the President's Council on Physical Fitness and Sports.
http://www.hoptechno.com/book11.htm

The Healthy Refrigerator
Heart-healthy eating tips for all ages.
http://www.healthyfridge.org

Shape Up America!
A national initiative to educate consumers about ways to maintain a healthy weight.
http://www.shapeup.org/

Cookbooks

American Heart Association. *American Heart Association Low-Fat, Low Cholesterol Cookbook*. 2nd edition. Times Books, 1998.

American Heart Association. *The New American Heart Association Cookbook: 25th Anniversary Edition*. Times Books, 1999.

Lakhani, Fatim. *Indian Recipes for a Healthy Heart: 140 Low-Fat, Low-Cholesterol, Low-Sodium Gourmet Dishes from India*. Fahil Publishing Company, 1992.

Lund, Joanna M. *The Heart Smart Healthy Exchanges Cookbook*. Perigee, 1999.

Ornish, Dean. *Eat More, Weigh Less: Dr. Dean Ornish's Advantage Ten Program for Losing Weight Safely While Eating Abundantly*. Revised edition. Quill, 2000.

Rippe, James M. and others. *The Healthy Heart Cookbook For Dummies®*. John Wiley & Sons, 2000.

General Health Information

HealthAtoZ.com
Patient-friendly health information that includes a large section on heart disease.
http://www.healthatoz.com

MEDLINEplus Medical Encyclopedia
An illustrated encyclopedia of diseases, tests, symptoms, and surgeries.
http://www.nlm.nih.gov/medlineplus/encyclopedia.html

The Merck Manual of Medical Information, Home Edition
An extensive online medical textbook for consumers.
http://www.merckhomeedition.com/home.html

Virtual Hospital
Includes information for patients on a broad range of health topics.
http://www.vh.org

Information on Alternative Therapies

American Association of Naturopathic Physicians
3201 New Mexico Avenue, NW, Suite 350
Washington, DC 20016
Tel: (202) 895–1392
Toll-free: 1–866–538–2267
General information about naturopathic medicine and finding a practitioner.
http://www.naturopathic.org/

American Association of Oriental Medicine
Lists licensed acupuncture practitioners by area.
http://www.aaom.org/

HealthWorld Online
Detailed information about numerous alternative therapies, fitness, and nutrition.
http://www.healthy.net

Whole Health MD
Combines alternative and complementary therapies with traditional medicine.
http://www.WholeHealthMD.com/

Personal Record

Primary Care Physician/Family Physican: **Phone #**

Cardiologist: **Phone #**

Pharmacy: **Phone #**

Allergies:

Current Medications (including complementary therapies and supplements)

Name of Medication	Purpose of Medication	Dose	How Often Taken Per Day (Circle One)	Date Started	Date Stopped
			1 2 3 4		
			1 2 3 4		
			1 2 3 4		
			1 2 3 4		
			1 2 3 4		
			1 2 3 4		
			1 2 3 4		
			1 2 3 4		

Continued over

Name of Medication	Purpose of Medication	Dose	How Often Taken Per Day (Circle One)	Date Started	Date Stopped
			1 2 3 4		
			1 2 3 4		
			1 2 3 4		
			1 2 3 4		
			1 2 3 4		
			1 2 3 4		

Heart Procedures	Date	Hospital
☐ *Echocardiogram*		
☐ *Exercise test*		
☐ *Heart cath*		
☐ *Angioplasty/Stent*		
☐ *Heart surgery*		

Symptoms

Date	Time	Symptom	Activity at the time of symptom	Duration	Severity on scale of 1 to 10 (1=mild, 10=severe)	What relieved your symptom?

Date	Time	Symptom	Activity at the time of symptom	Duration	Severity on scale of 1 to 10 (1=mild, 10=severe)	What relieved your symptom?

Rehabilitation Clinic/Other Wellness Center Contact Information

Name and Address	Contact Phone Number	Fax	Email

Questions I would like to ask my doctor or nurse

Notes

Notes

Notes

index

References to figures: *3fig*
references to tables: *119t*
references to More Detail boxes in bold: **4**
references to Key Point boxes in bold italic: ***5***
references to Self-Help boxes in italic: *12*